D1600529

THAT FIRST BITE

Karen Rose

PaperJacks LTD.

TORONTO   NEW YORK

PaperJacks

THAT FIRST BITE:
Journal of a Compulsive Overeater

PaperJacks LTD

330 STEELCASE RD. E., MARKHAM, ONT. L3R 2M1
210 FIFTH AVE., NEW YORK, N.Y. 10010

Pomerica Press edition published 1979

PaperJacks edition published July 1987

ISBN 0-7701-0647-1

To Beth H., Jean S., Doris S., and all my other anonymous but glorious friends in OA,
I dedicate this book

How much easier it would be if there were only visible events to describe rather than invisible transformations.
William Irwin Thompson

Part One

Gaining

I was a skinny kid.

In Brooklyn in P.S. 161, in the fourth grade, they wanted to put me in the health room. When I went down to look at this health room (the rear of the nurse's office) I saw puny children napping. I went home and stated that I was not puny and unhealthy. My parents agreed with me and we won that battle. I remained in the fourth grade, open to fractions, Thomas Jefferson, and fighting for first in line.

"Skinny brat," people called me who wanted to hurt my feelings. And they did. Especially when I got to thirteen and was still "skinny." But by 14 I was coming along nicely and did not have to worry about my body, breasts, legs, or weight until I was in my thirties.

I had no idea that such a body was a gift. I had no idea that it could change. From the time I was five I had one friend who was obese — our mothers talked even then about getting her weight off — but I never could understand why it mattered. Nor, except for noting that people often hurt her by mean remarks, did I think of her fatness at all. She was my friend.

My thing was just not "fatness." It was the nature of the universe that had a tendency to do me in. At fifteen I'd sunk into despondency but never told anyone except the boy downstairs. He was much older and in college and therefore might be in a position to help; and he was also very handsome and strong. He did help. He showed me a quote in his Abnormal Psych book that explained that many people suffered depressions in adolescence. He talked to me for days, smoking his pipe, being gentle, and knowing everything. I got well.

By seventeen, myself in college, I had another depression. And the depression this time was such that I stood at the end of the IRT line at Brooklyn College and looked down and knew that if I stayed there one more day I would throw myself in front of a train. I knew that I would do this. And it scared me, so I went home and got into bed. The boy from downstairs came up, but this time he couldn't help me. I saw clearly that if I were not depressed, I would love him, but I could not break through the sullen, sunken air all about me. He went downstairs and I went to a psychiatrist.

"Go west," the doctor said. "Get away from home." I had by now settled upon the Grand Theme of my depressions, and this theme dealt, it seemed to me, not with geography at all, but with the subjects of death, existentialism, and the true nature of reality. But I went west and it did help.

I got a job, started college four nights a week, and would settle everything by majoring in philosophy.

I turned eighteen and was to give a paper in front of my class dealing with Immanuel Kant's work. The boy from downstairs arrived, met me after class with a stuffed bear. We named the bear Immanuel and married shortly thereafter.

We came back from a disastrous honeymoon and found a telegram under the door from the Turkish Government. My husband had applied to teach in Turkey ages before he'd even finished his Master's in English. He'd forgotten about the application and here was the job.

We set off for Konya, the home of the whirling dervishes, and ended up spending the year in Istanbul instead. This was to be a miserably unhappy year for both of us and I got fat. Looking back now, I remember eating all the time, but then there was nothing else to do. If you're really not too happy with someone, you can always eat together. Finally, at last, having stayed far too long, I admitted defeat and left.

I don't even remember dieting. Suddenly I was thin again. And no weight problem until now — a now that started about three years before this Journal. Depressions became manageable: it turns out everybody has them, and with the help of antidepressants here and there — "there" usually being at the end of a long-term romance — they went away.

But the weight problem, which I first thought of as the ordinary ups and downs I've watched everybody go through, came but did not, this time, go away. By the time I began this Journal, I weighed 140 pounds, having been up to 160 and down and up in the previous years, and before I could come to terms with the whole thing I hit 200. I'm five-two.

I got heavier than my father, who had always been called the trite "Mr. Five-by-Five," and heavier than my brother (and somehow one know instinctively that a kid sister should never weigh more than her worshiped, handsome, and well-built brother).

I could not believe how big my pants had to be. Holding them open, looking down into the Grand Canyon of them, I could never believe I would fill them. But I filled them. Size 40 pants. Size 44 blouses.

When I started this Journal, two years ago, I taught elementary school, took care of my dog, Annie, and my cat, Katharine Hepburn, and ate. The rest of my life — thin friends, lovers, books, writing, theater, play — all of it was rapidly vanishing. Food.

The life of a compulsive is cyclic. I feel so little desire to date the items in this Journal. For so long now, weeks and months have merely been patterns of eating and trying not to eat. A compulsive overeater moves slowly except toward food. Yet one continues to notice the calendar.

(1)

October 20, 1975

It always begins, the diet, with a *before* or an *after*. Before the return to a place where nobody's seen you fat. Before an annual big family celebration where they haven't seen you *this* fat. You're a year fatter.

Or after a binge of greater and more frightening proportions than ever. Today I begin *after*. I'm so sick from overeating I think I am dying. Yesterday, which was, of course, only the culmination of four weeks of excruciating eating, I ate (at school where supposedly I am an adult teaching children): a bear claw, scrambled eggs, leftover sandwiches. I was already so sick I didn't eat at recess. By lunch I was still sick to my stomach, but I ate:

    pizza
    fruit cocktail
    Jello mold
    more leftover sandwiches
    fruit cake
    ice cream

PL, one of the teachers, looked at me eating, and by a throat-clearing and a gaze that took it all in — me, the food, the accumulation of days of such eating (witnessed by them all, increasing since September at which time I was already 15 pounds heavier than when we'd waved our June good-byes) — tried to tell me not to eat.

I continued eating, wondering what I could get more of. And then PL said, "Karen, you don't really need that." I glared at her and said, "Only Joyce has that job." Then PL said, pointing to still another teacher a ways down the long cafeteria table we eat at, "Don't blame me. Zena told me to try to stop you."

All this across the table, in front of the men, in front of everyone, and all in a jocular manner. I laughed it off. They are nice people and mean me no harm.

I die when something like that happens.

Joyce walked out with me when the bell rang. "Sometimes I hate them," she said.

"Yeah."

(2)

It is safe lying here in the bedroom, trees against my window. Late at night is quiet, a writing time. Milk on the bedstand beside me. Ms. Hepburn dips an occasional tongue into the milk but she knows it is mine.

I am either fasting or just on milk to help settle my stomach. I am not only sick to my stomach but am having a heart attack. Or asphyxiation. That's a possibility. My wall heater gives off a persistent smell of poisoningness. Or maybe H., my next-door neighbor, is painting his apartment again. More likely it's my wall heater out to get me. Maybe the girl next door is committing suicide. But I don't know her well enough to knock on her door. It could be suicide — she gets a lot of parking tickets.

It is not safe here. What I really need to do is get out of here. I'll just hop out for a bite to eat.

(3)

Be thankful for:

1. It's legal to eat. Nobody but your doctor is out to stop you.
2. You're not an alcoholic. If you drank as overmuch as you eat, you'd be dead by now.
3. It's not a heroin addiction. You couldn't afford it. This way for only an extra $100 a month you can support your habit.
4. You don't have to depend on anybody else to eat with. It's perfectly fine to be alone on a binge.
5. You always have something to do.
6. You won't die of senility. You won't live that long.
7. You can immediately spot others like yourself. Those with your disease.
8. Gives you an opportunity to keep buying the latest fashions. And there are enough department stores in town to spread the debts around.
9. Other women like you immediately. You're to be pitied and encouraged. You are no threat to them. They will often tell you that you really look fine.

(4)

October 24
Piece of Pizza Scene: One-Act Play
Time: Approximately three times a week, a little after the dinner-crowd rush.
Place: Selected Piece of Pizza restaurants anywhere in the greater Los Angeles area.
Treatment: Comedic. To be accompanied by light-hearted music.

I have so arranged it that I will have Katharine Hepburn in my car, meowing in her traveling kit, and Annie on the leash. Thus when I arrive at the Piece of Pizza place I have already set up punishment. It will be clearly impossible to get a combination dinner for two (for one) home safely with all the clutter in the car.

"Big pizza with the rest of the stuff, lady?"

"Oh, no, the snack size, please. The $2.95 one."

I had hoped he wouldn't ask and just give me the big one. Maybe he remembers me from before, though I don't remember him, and maybe he's figured out what my story is. "Oh, no, the snack size, please." Shit. Plus two cokes. Two small ones, for me and my combination.

I get the food into the car. Close to me. I will drive with my left hand, my right balancing the pizza box and the spaghetti and salad plastic containers against the cat carrier which is wedged under the glove compartment between the front seat and the dashboard. Annie drools in the back.

The dog's silent saliva dripping is not unnoticed by the mad driver. I must have a piece of the pizza NOW — while it's still hot.

Red light. Edge top open, one eye on light. Eat piece, forget to give dog bite. Take another piece, remember to give small bite to dog. Cat meowing but unreachable — even I couldn't open the cat carrier in the car.

I pride myself on carrying a lot of things at one time; prodigious packages rise upward in my magical arrangements. Of course, I drop a lot of things, but I usually go for the gamble. I want to make it up the stairs in one trip. Because I must eat instantly upon opening the door of the apartment. I try not to notice that I am vile enough to have considered leaving the cat alone in the car (after all, she'd be safe). I'll get my whole family and the restaurant up the stairs.

Meanwhile, back at the car, in my purse, which is large (similar to a grocery bag in all but color and stamina), the cokes have leaked. Spaghetti sauce and coke are also infiltrating the library books on the seat of the car. I get to pay for a lot of library books.

I make it upstairs and I go in and eat it all.

And will probably have to go out for dessert.

I'll go alone without the animals.

Maybe I'll be attacked and killed. On a full stomach. You know what people say? They say, don't have it in the house. That's the secret of dieting. Don't have it in the house.

I just figured out why I no longer enjoy taking a bath. It used to be my favorite form of relaxation. And I used to brush my teeth three times a day. Now I find myself needing to remind myself to bathe, to brush my teeth. Suddenly (for as well as Obese, I have grown Obtuse), I know why I've lost my love of the clean taste and clear skin. Mirrors.

(5)

Obesity is a uniquely human problem. Blame the brain — not because of mysterious psychological reasons . . . but because the new brain — the neocortex — has overruled the appetite and satiety centers in the old brain for so long that they no longer signal the body's needs.

In the obese and in the millions who are fighting encroaching overweight, the desire to eat apparently originates in the visual cortex rather than in the primitive hunger centers. For example, French researchers found that obese subjects who had been loaded with glucose still found the sweet taste of sucrose pleasant. Normally, the sweet taste would become sickening. Somehow the natural satiating mechanism has been subverted in the obese. . . .

Electrical stimulation of the brain's hunger center will produce a raging appetite, even if the subject has just stuffed down an enormous meal.

—Marilyn Ferguson, *The Brain Revolution*

That's me, a little old electrical stimulator.

(6)

A friend: The problem is you eat too much.
Me: Well, I know, but that's not exactly the problem.
Friend: I have watched you eat too much.
Another friend: Take salt with you wherever you go. It's as simple as a lack of salt sometimes.
Me: I'll take salt.

(7)

I can only write about yesterday because I've been awake 30 minutes and *good* so far. I want to write to Webster and have them add another meaning to their list of definitions of "good:" "Not bingeing voraciously on calorific food." Yesterday I ate, in order:

9:00 a.m.	Egg McMuffin, orange juice, jelly
1:00 p.m.	Quarter-pounder, French fries, shake
2:30 p.m.	10 caramels
	1 pt. chocolate ice cream 1 pt. vanilla
	½ an angel food cake
	Swiss cheese
	2 real Pepsies
6:00 p.m.	Crab Newburgh Fruit salad
10:00 p.m.	Rest of angel food cake, ice cream, spaghetti, 10 caramels. From 8 to 9:30 I sat at a school meeting and pretended to be sane. Probably everybody there thought I was sane. I'm very effective at teaching reading, and though I look grotesque from the outside, it doesn't seem to hurt the reading scores.

(8)

Today I ate two eggs and three ounces of cheese at about 1. I am on a diet today. The sleep is upon me. I want an apple. I am afraid to have an apple. I might get much worse and binge. Today it is my intention to be OA (Overeater Anonymous — I went there but it wasn't for me, but they sure are right about compulsive being compulsive). One bit of the wrong stuff will kill me. To give up sweets for life. The only way to go. I weigh 150 pounds. Another size up. I'm almost out of the "larges." That's incredible. I do not want to go on living. I believe it's nonsense for me to feel this way.

Sleeping is really great, though. And I don't eat when I sleep. I'll try fasting Saturday and Sunday.

Same evening: Very depressed. Everything bleak as could be. Went to N's. Ate dinner but did not badly overeat. Ate approximately 1500 calories today. It was worth the suffering of the day to have had a day where I wasn't driven compulsively.

I'll meet some people when this is all over — this fatness.

(9)

Binge.

(10)

Ten days later

A while since the last entry. One can write out of suffering, but not out of despair.

First it was not despair. I was controlling the eating and I got into the crazy kind of hope that hits me every time I am sane for as much as four days. I am convinced I am cured. I'll be thin again and can walk with other women.

After four days of dieting — whether I've lost only 3 pounds, as in this case, or 8 pounds, as in some cases — I am relieved of many problems:

1. Clothing: there is the hope I won't have to buy anything new — "new" means "larger" — this week. If I lose

weight I have a continually new wardrobe at my command, right out of my own closets, all things I could wear a week or so before I was too big. Intelligence would dictate I buy a larger size and "grow into it." That is, intelligence based on experience. Economic feasibility. No.

2. The pain in my chest stops. This pain is variously attributed to the heart or sometimes other causes. Esophagitis?

3. A delay in the breaking through of the walls of my chest by enormous backing up of food I've eaten.

4. Heartburn from overeating goes away after three days of sensible eating.

5. Various lower-end problems, too embarrassing to discuss, are all cured in three days, and the aches in my arms and body lessen.

All this and promises of a golden more to come in the land of the thin and the free.

And I blew it on the fifth day by eating a mixture of sweet potatoes, pineapple, and apples. Sugar.

Fantastic. "I'll just have a little more, please." My hostess, a parent who volunteers in my reading program, has seen me gain the weight and is worried over me — always pushing her hypnotist, or her latest pills, or the Exercise of the Month — is, of course, trapped from the beginning. If she serves an all-protein dinner to her whole family, naturally I'll feel guilty. So there is chicken, deliciously prepared, for me, and a beautiful salad, and a vegetable. And just that one goody for them. No dessert.

And if I ask for some? Just a little — well, maybe just a little more — can she say no? It sits there, casseroled, its aroma a magnetic force yanking me to it.

We're both trapped in my gluttony. I am a fool and a coward and an idiot of the highest order. I will never get to a swimming pool. There will never be another man worth having, my arteries will swell, and I will continue to have my friends hate me for my failures and I will hate them for being normal. "Just a little bit more, please. It's so good."

Psychodynamically this all means I am a shithead now and ever will be one.

(11)

The casserole recedes into the belly of yesterday and I am evermore again on the way to Baskin-Robbins and McDonald's and Winchells. On the way home on Sunset last night I passed the UCLA Homecoming festivities. Lights and turning wheels filled my rear-view mirror. The brightest-lit Ferris wheel of all time, surely. Moving slowly, happily, eternally, a combination of lighted geodesic dome patterns and joie de vivre.

Lately I only see things through rear-view mirrors.

(12)

Grits, Spanish omelette, cinnamon bread, peanut butter, cookies, hamburger, salad, ice-cream sandwich, double Baskin-Robbins (cherry and Rocky Road), chicken and rice, asparagus, lemon squares, peanut butter and peach preserves, open-faced, two sandwiches, calories 2800, a low day.

(13)

My big romance so far this year is with George. He is an alcoholic but doesn't admit it. We go to this restaurant where you get a complete dinner and two drinks each for some convenient price. He drinks my drinks and I eat his desserts. A hot and heavy romance. Would either of us notice if the other wasn't there?

(14)

Proverbs for Compulsive Eaters

If it's in the house, you're going to eat it.
If it's not in the house, you're going to go out and get it and then eat it.

———————

It's our life against the surcease of a piece of cheesecake.

———————

Fat girls are very good on the telephone.

———————

Fat girls have lots of shoes.

———————

I'm sick unto death, but if you could just bring me a little something to eat.

———————

The only diet that even stands a chance for the compulsive eater begins the night before, never the morning after.

———————

Even hoping becomes part of the state of despair.

———————

It is no longer unfashionable for a woman to steal, stand up for her rights, join the football team. She could probably even rape someone. The only thing that's unfeminine is to be fat.

_____

Possession seems the most probable cause. But who will by my exorcist?

(15)

November 10, '77

A man in my life. We met in the Bodhi Tree, in front of the incense and prayer beads. He had Castaneda under his arm and was gently fingering an Indian string of beads. I thought he was looking at me but couldn't believe it. He spoke to me about incense. I answered him about incense. And there we were. Then he said, "Are you happy?" I'd been suicidal all day. "Right now, I am," I said. He asked me out.

Why would a handsome, attractive, intelligent man ask me out at this point in my life? Before the fat, yes, they did. But now, when he doesn't even know that once I was attractive? Maybe he thinks I'll be an easy lay. Fat girls appreciate you more.

Not one to be able to live comfortably with big questions, I asked him on our first date (he had a salad and I had cheesecake, right in front of him), "Doesn't it bother you that I'm fat?"

He said it didn't. He went on about it quite a bit. He explained that sex he could have with anyone. There had to be more to a girl. I might be on the problem side physiologically but soulwise I was okay. He practically provided illustrations along with the mysticism.

If it's a line, I'm glad he's thrown it to me.

One thing about fat girls. We're the grateful type. I didn't eat again tonight.

(16)

Once when I was thin I dated a man who was far too heavy. But he was fascinating, and good to be with. Nothing came of it because he felt I was worthless if I would go out with him. Only if I had something wrong with me would I date him. Now I have met Steven and I hesitate to see him. I mean something must be wrong with him if he'd go out with someone who looks like this.

(17)

Steven brought William Erwin Thompson and Jonas Salk to dinner tonight. I figure I can control the food better if we eat here. So I make steak, baked potatoes, biscuits. A man has to eat. He's not, in fact, much of an eater. He is thirsty for talk. I want to know if he'd go to bed with me. I can't even think about whether I want to go to bed with him — that's hardly relevant when I'm this ugly.

One part of mankind wishes to take us into rockets, computers, and a cultural unity that comes from computerized medicine, computerized music, poetry, and film, and cybernetic organisms in which the education of the mind is achieved by hooking up the cells of the brain directly to teaching machines. The other part of mankind is struggling to develop consciousness so as to obviate the need for machines. If one has *pratyahara* (yogic control of the senses), he has no need of drugs; if one has *kriya* (control of the central nervous system), he has no need of computers; if one has *samadhi* (cosmic consciousness), he has no need of moon rockets; for it is the characteristic of an infinite space that all the points are equidistant from one another, and so one does not have to get anywhere if he is at his own center.

— William Erwin Thompson

The talk is good. I ended by telling him about my interest in doing a book on the brain and meditation. He looked at me like how could I have had access to all that stuff and not changed my life. Or maybe he didn't look at me that way at all.

How the hell could I have had access to everything I've had and not changed my life?

He went home pretty early.

(18)

I was on the way to meet Steven. Splitting-apart sensation. Eat something, *kindala*. Hamburger and shake.

Stunkard, in 1959 ... analyzed eating patterns and described two as pathologic, the "Night Eating Syndrome" and the "Binge Eating Syndrome." ... He describes the Binge Eating Syndrome as characterized by the sudden, compulsive ingestion of very large amounts of food in a very short time, usually with subsequent agitation and self-condemnation. It too represents a reaction to stress, ... tends to be closely linked to specific precipitating circumstances.

— Hilde Bruch, *Eating Disorders*

Damn the psychologists. I, the Syndrome, felt better. Had I met a narcissistic need? A masochistic need? I can't win against psychology and god knows I've listened to

it in a worshiping position, my belly groveling on the
ground beneath me. Sometimes, just sometimes, let me
trust myself. I feel better after the food and my blood
sugar is raised and I will be better with Steven.

(19)

Level of sexual fantasy. Huge globs of flesh welcomed
by eager arms. All his life he's waited for you. He carries
Rubens Miniature Art Library in his pocket. "You are
beautiful, my dearest. Voluptuous."

(20)

In regard to my romance with Steven I seem to be
past the fantasy stage, though memories of it perk inside
of me. My head plays a recording with Maurice Chevalier
singing, "I remember it well." But what can I fantasize
with any new man? I am too old, if not too fat, to see
it all laid out before me as I used to — a touch of Cinderella
here, a touch of Elizabeth Taylor there, a touch of magic
wishwash here, Beauty and the Beast there.

Normally by now I'd have the children named. The
date and hour of our disclosures of panting hunger for
each other planned — "Oh, did you? You did?" I would
be talking about nothing but Steven to my friends.

I told Joyce at recess that I thought it was total old
age and she said, no, it was more like growing up.

Maybe it is because Beauty can afford both fantasy
and the luxury of multitudinous choices of repetitive fantasies. And Beast can't.

(21)

Even the children at school see the weight gain. I am

approached on yard duty, by one of Joyce's fourth-graders, "Miss R, are you pregnant?"

"Hah, hah," I say. "A Miss can't get pregnant [Modern Pedagogy 101 and Women's Lib 102 have left me untouched]. You know that."

"Oh, yes, she can. You know she can."

"Well, don't," I say and walk off, briskly busy. I have the next child I see bring me a package of cookies from the cafeteria. (Don't tell them who they're for, I want to shout after him. But I don't. How can you expect a seven-year-old to be an effective cover agent?)

(22)

I'm afraid to go out to dinner with Steven. That I'll slip and eat and damn myself. And of course that's no image a girl wants to have, right?

But suddenly I realize that if I'm honest with him — unsexy as it is — if I tell him I'm not charming and buoyant and happy and into a of lot things, but basically morose and into food, and if we don't become lovers — that's okay too. If I'm with him as I am, instead of as I want to be, and I lose him, *then that will have been our relationship.*

(23)

I was honest. He says he doesn't think I'm morose.

(24)

He hasn't called in a week. With the holidays coming this isn't a good sign.

(25)

I'm morose. And burgeoning.

(26)

The obese do not have free thought patterns.

Matter is a passing stage of spirit.
— Jack Schwarz, via Marilyn Ferguson

(27)

I took my parents to a funeral today of a friend from the post office where my father worked before he retired. I didn't know the man and found myself listening intently to every word of the service. Perhaps because it was an unfamiliar service, or perhaps because I was not emotionally involved in a personal grief, I heard it all so clearly.

Some things are beginning to sneak in on me. Stuff I could easily live without. So help me I don't know where it's coming from. Seepage.

> For whosoever shall find his life shall lose it;
> and whosoever will lose his life for my sake shall
> find it.

Matthew 16:25

If you grow up Jewish, encounters with Jesus are mind-blowing. There are no old, mixed-up notions. You hear what he said same as you'd hear what any individual says. This is far scarier than knowing full well that no man ever rose up from the dead and that the kids across the street believe that the man hanging there is really the son of God. It gets scary, the whole subject, and I mostly just pray it will go away quickly and quietly.

(28)

Thanksgiving

I ate everything on the table, in the refrigerator, and was into pumpkin chip cookies in my sister-in-law's refrigerator.

(29)

December 10
I have been dieting and I will not stop because I am not hearing from Steven. The days are long. I remember how days passed in movies I saw when I was a kid. Magic-like, the pages of the calendar turned and magic-like the seasons changed, and quickly the desired date was reached. The problem was solved by the good intentions and labor of the lady who lived through the calendar-turning days. But somebody somewhere seems to think I must live each day all the way through, flat out, just like that, the rough parts blatant, no quarter given for intention and desire.

Perhaps I am coming out of a seizure. A certain shift in my consciousness can be felt. Maybe I can avoid the next binge for several hours — maybe

Have been hanging in there. Maybe I could develop anorexia for a year or two.

"My dear, you should eat something. You're disappearing."

"It isn't healthy to be so thin."

(30)

Ten days of model conduct. Eight pounds off. This time isn't as hard as other times have been. Funny. There are no rhymes, no reasons.

(31)

There's a piece of cake in my refrigerator. How did it get there??? Angel food. Well, I *must* eat it. If I don't eat it, it will feel like a failure in life. Somebody made that cake with the intent for it to be eaten. It has a certain karma, and I, too, who have now come upon it. It has always been destined to culminate in my refrigerator.

From Earl Ubell, author of *How to Save Your Life:*
"Can't Diet or Exercise — or Break Habits? 'Behaviorism' offers This Key to a New You."

> You want to lose weight and you eat. . . You
> want and you can't. You're not alone — millions
> of men and women are trapped by their killing
> habit. Take eating. Americans are 15% over-
> weight and it is killing us with heart attacks. Yet
> eating too much is a habit. If you want to live
> longer you have to change the habit. . .
>   Then a strange thing happened. I was over-
> weight. I thought of dying. I thought of my father
> on his deathbed — overweight. Every time I went
> for the high-calorie food, I saw the picture of
> my dad!

Mr. Ubell goes on to explain that all you need to do
is apply a little Skinner here and there. If you punish
a behavior just before it happens, then the chances are
that the behavior will not be repeated.

To set up the punishment, all you have to do is list
the foods you don't want to eat and think of an unpleasant
scene before you eat them. You will soon be turning away
from that food. Soon the behavior stops before it starts.

First of all, I think it's morally revolting to use the
death of a family member in that manner. Second, any
healthy, decent compulsive eater can eat at his father's
deathbed and make plans for catering of the funeral!

(32)

Diary with Voices

— Well, I'll get some dinner.
— You're not even hungry.

— Yeah, but I feel a cold coming on. I'll just get a hamburger and shake.

— Illness, crap. You're a glutton. Illness — possibly an excuse. But this is gluttony. You can get a hamburger and a coke.

Out we go!

"Quarter-pounder with cheese and a chocolate shake, please."

My god, it's like a mantra.

(33)

Does the transition to the other being, the compulsive giant, who eats into the core of the universe, occur at night? How can I prevent it from happening? What can I do that I haven't done before? It's tricky to have to learn to outguess your own self. I feel like all of my "I"s are in a football huddle waiting for instructions on how to break through the lines and capture the ball. It's a question of throwing to me, without interception by that one particular player "I" who cheats, commands, and kills. Anything for a touchdown.

(34)

There is a constant self-monitoring. I try to figure out the links. I want to believe it's physical and when I do not eat I try to see why. Tonight my car broke down in traffic and the cop couldn't have been nastier. But I did not eat. Why? Adrenalin in the blood as the result of anger changing the chemistry, or the expression of anger at the policeman, changing the psychology? But there is no psychology without chemistry. If my blood were like that all the time, would I be able to diet? Oh, hypothalamus, who art thou?

. . . The appestat which regulates the quantity

of food that is eaten must have a cellular basis; the indications are that the primary mechanism is located in the hypothalamus of the brain. These nerve cells require nourishment and it is possible — indeed highly probable, in my opinion — that obesity is often a disease of deficient nutrition, that is, poor nutrition of the nervous tissues involved in the control of food consumption. It is possible that this poor nutrition dates back to early childhood or earlier and that individuals who tend strongly to be obese have had their appetite mechanism more or less permanently deranged by bad nutrition.

— Roger Williams, *Nutrition in a Nutshell*

(I do have to admit that my mother could never get me to drink my milk.)

(35)

Existence will remain meaningless for you if you yourself do not penetrate into it — with active love and if you do not in this way discover its meaning for yourself. Everything is waiting to be hallowed by you; it is waiting for this meaning to be disclosed and to be realized by you. Meet the world with the fullness of your being and you shall meet God. If you wish to believe, Love.

— Martin Buber

(36)

Recommendations from Fat Girl on
Certain Fat Subjects

Letter to Baskin-Robbins franchise: How to Handle Compulsives:

Do not ever say: "Say, weren't you in a few minutes ago? With the double scoop?"

Remarks I have promised myself never to make and which, so far, I have never made:

At dinner table, as hostess offers food around for the last time:

"Here, give it to me. Old Garbage Can here will eat it." and

"Of course I eat a lot. Why else would I look like a van?"

Notes on reorganization of Lane Bryant and other shops specializing in clothing for fat girls:

Only fat salesgirls. Stop putting those damned skinny models in the windows. Who are you fooling? We know the dress won't look like that on us. We pay double for clothes that have less style than Woolworth stuff which anybody normal can get for next to nothing. And the people on the street know about Lane Bryant. It kills me to even have the Charge-a-Plate in my wallet. Also get rid of the tall girls' section. They're tall, beautiful, skinny, a sexual fantasy to legions of men. Get them and their damned long-sleeved blouses out of here. Get rid of the entire tall, thin business.

I do not want to shop with normal people.

Report of in-depth study of Jean Nidetch's Weight Watchers organization:

Fuck tuna fish.

(38)

Six hours of freedom from the compulsion produces such an intense change in being that it must be due to divine intervention.

(39)

"Joyce, I can't go into that classroom."

"Yeah, you can."

"I'm insane."

"So are the kids. You belong together."

"I have to stop eating for one hour and twenty minutes if I go in there."

"You'll make it. And come this afternoon and do a creative writing lesson."

"I'll teach them naming ice cream flavors."

"Great. We have a present for you."

The present turns out to be a bag of tennis balls her class has collected for Annie.

(40)

I've just eaten eight pieces of pizza, one quart of really lousy spaghetti, and now I want to kill myself. The shame and horror is unending, unceasing.

The mere discomfort of the body is irrelevant.

I am hanging on the question of whether or not to go to Baskin-Robbins. I will. I always lose. The debate debates and I think I, whoever that is, am in there fighting, but I always go.

Rendezvous at B & R

First I drive to all the spots within a 15-minute radius to see which has the shortest line. Taking a number is not the number one spectator sport of a compulsive overeater.

Why are there so many people here? What's wrong with them? And so many of them thin. Damn.

Number 6. What do I do from now until then? I have rapidly read all 31 flavors. I have counted on such items as Charlie Brownie, Pralines and Cream, Blueberry Birth Miasma, B&R Diabetes Prize Flavor Nuts, and Toads with Fudge Ribbon.

Number 6 at last.

"Yes, ma'm."

"We'll have 12 ounces of Rocky Road, 12 ounces of Pralines and Cream — gee, is Cha Cha Charoom good?"

"Want to taste it?"

"Give me a cone while you're making up that other stuff."

He makes the cone.

He repeats my order: "Is that it?"

"No, just start. I need to remember what they all want. Also, do you have a Banana Split Pie?"

"No, you need to order those in advance now."

"Oh, put in a Mud Pie then."

(I will not order in advance. I'm going to be finished with this eating thing soon. Yet I remember that I have heard that drunks on Antabuse have to stop taking the medicine five days in advance not to get ill when they drink, and they plan it that way. Five days consigned to not changing your state of consciousness.)

"Do you have any Fudge Brownies?"

"Sure."

"Give me two of those and a chocolate ice cream sandwich."

"Okay."

I hand him my teacher's paycheck and we call it even.

I see myself in the swinging polished door of the shop as I leave. Whose are those big hips and that bag of ice cream?

I take it home to all of us.

(41)

There is pain in every ounce I wear, every arm I carry.

(42)

I am not going to get up and eat the spaghetti. I want

the spaghetti because I saw the tomato sauce. Visual cues, as they say. I wasn't even thinking of spaghetti before.

(43)

I'll do anything but stop eating.

(44)

I want to be dead.

(45)

Compulsive fact: Eat fewer calories than you burn and you'll lose weight. Carbohydrates, fat, be damned. Work it any way, just work it, and you'll lose weight. There really is little need for "researching" the problem.
But we are the desperate,
The ones ad creators love.
We'll buy Ayds,
   machines,
   scales to the half-ounce
   pregnant urine
   grapefruit
   kelp
   cyanide
We are not stupid but we will buy all that and read every ad in every Sunday's paper, and every monthly *Reader's Digest*. Perhaps we are doing something wrong, maybe we didn't read all the directions right. Perhaps there is something we don't know.
We are the desperate.

> . . . not even the most dedicated food freak has
> yet suggested that a good helping of fried cod
> or a slice of pizza can produce an instant boost
> in IQ. But now researchers at the MIT have dis-

covered that individual meals do indeed have an immediate effect on some aspects of the brain's activity. The findings involved serotonin, which is one of the four or five chemicals in the brain known as neurotransmitters. . . . Serotonin itself . . . works in control sleep, food consumption, carbohydrate meals raise serotonin.

— *Newsweek,* November 27, 1972

A statement like that, thrown loosely into my mixed mind, tends to blow it.

(46)

Today I am willing to eat. I'll approach it intelligently. I'd like a lox brunch. Don't feel like ice cream yet. Feel willing to have some cheese. Cheese will be my salvation.

Who wants to eat today? *(sung solo)*

(Chorus) I do.

Who wants to diet today? *(solo)*

(Chorus) I do.

I do. I don't. I do, I don't. *(single voices and chorus refrains)*

Mirror, mirror, on the wall, who's the fattest of them all?

(47)

Not only do your thighs no longer allure, but they rub together, meshed in flesh, and they hurt like hell, all the time, rubbing and rubbing and reminding and reminding. You pig.

(48)

The preliminary movement of Rajayoga is a careful self-discipline by which good habits of

mind are substituted for the lawless movements
that indulge the lower nervous being. By the practice of truth, by renunciation of all forms of ego-
istic seeking, by abstention from injury to others,
by purity, by constant meditation and inclination
to the divine Purusha who is the true lord of
the mental kingdom, a *pure, glad clear state of
mind* and heart is established. This is the first
step only. . . .

— Sri Aurobindo

He's got me down there all right: "lawless movements
that indulge the lower nervous being."
I doubt the pure, glad clear state of mind is coming
to me soon. With every bite of Aurobindo, I stuff in
sugar cookies.

(49)

When I was in my twenties I swam nude in the Little
Sur River with the poet Eric Barker. We laughed and
laughed, at the unmistakable beauty of the bodies we
had been given. That is the truth. I swear to it. Eric wrote
in a book he gave me, "To the water nymph of the swimming hole." And I cried over his poetry.

A Philosopher

Though they took the trees away
And locked him in his room,
Nothing could break that green allegiance!
When I went to see him
He was sitting very quiet, looking
At his painting. It was called "The Wood."
But even one tree had given him shade enough

To hide the naked walls and wind enough
To blow the ceiling off!

"They're with me all the time," he said,
"Just thinking on the one
Has brought the whole grove in."

Last week I saw an old boy friend enter the theater
where I was seeing the Jung films. I missed the last fifteen
minutes of the film so that there would be no chance
of his seeing me at the end of the movie. I was long
gone by then. That too is the truth.

It's going past me now. The skinny-hipped girls are
waving their assy flags and the world is going past me
now.

(50)

— I really don't feel like eating anything.
    I go to the ice box, take out banana bread.

— You must eat it.
——— Why must I?
— You just must.

The banana bread is not good. It is not. I don't even
like it. I swat Ms. Hepburn away. It is all for me.

I eat it but I don't want to eat. What can I do? This
over and over againness. Now I want pizza. I'll try med-
itating on it. Antibehaviorist theory. No theory has ever
succeeded in making me want less. There is only *more*
in my vocabulary. I can't fail more than I do. I can only
FAIL AGAIN.

Cut out pictures of pizza and hang them up all over
the room. Why not? If the suggestion of food is not to
be overcome, how can you ever watch TV?

(51)

I have been reading about compulsives. Our stories are the same. Repeated failures. Suicide, though we consider it quite frequently while in the eating stage, is unlikely as long as we can keep eating. Eating has the advantage of (1) keeping us from suicide by further repressing whatever it is we are repressing, and (2) meeting our enormous death wish by being in itself a form of suicide, for we see, clearly, feel in our aches and our exhaustions and in the pains in our arms and the terrifying beating of our hearts that our health is being RUINED; as surely as an alcoholic liver there goes our heart, our arteries, and our saturated blood. How can you have (1) and (2) both? If you couldn't have, indeed, if you didn't demand (1) and (2) both, and then (3), (4), (5), and then (6), you wouldn't be a compulsive eater. If you only had a few numbers running, you might be a thin person who does commit suicide, or, if you also have hypoglycemia, you might be a murderer, or a vicious mother, or something equally romantic.

(52)

Fasting: Research and Practice Thereof

I know perfectly well that a person can fast away his fat with no danger because a plane crashed in the Arctic with a man and an overweight girl. When rescued, she looked great. Thirty pounds less. Had drunk snow. That rescue-adventure routine — they'll probably make a movie out of it.

I barely even know where the Arctic is. Can you get reservations? A chartered plane maybe. Me and twelve fat friends. Set us down, promise to return thirty days later, bearing size 12 bathing suits (and hot chocolates). The photographers will come. Maybe even Hugh Hefner.

All doctors' reports indicated that she was the healthier for the experience. So, no matter what the pros and cons are, or, more particularly, the cons which you hear from AMA spokesmen, I know it can be done with no danger to the health. And what the hell is a little danger anyway? Some statistics say that for every extra five pounds you gain you lose a year of life. Me for the cold snows.

Day 1. This is serious. Not a short, jumped-into thing. This one is serious. I am staying home from school. As I reach school something takes over and it is in constant demand of food to comfort itself for the hours ahead. I'll have to live with the guilt of not working. I have to break this eating pattern.

12 a.m. — first day. I feel lousy. Why? It can't be from not eating. It would take me two weeks on a foodless desert island to even get hungry. I'm reading a book on fasting by Paul Bragg. He's one of those health nuts who is completely healthy. Far older already than us fat folks will live to be he climbs mountains and crosses deserts. He hiked across Death Valley, California, to show that he didn't need salt during extremely hot weather. Salt is not one of my binge foods but something about Bragg captures the imagination:

> . . . I hired ten husky young college athletes to make the hike . . . a distance of approximately 30 miles. . . . I had no salt and on that 30 mile hike, I fasted. The hike was started at the end of July, . . .the thermometer stood at 105 degrees, . . .a dry hot heat, that seemed to want to melt you. . . .The college boys gobbled the salt tablets and guzzled quarts of cool water. . . .At lunch they ate ham sandwiches, drank cola drinks, and cheese sandwiches. . . . Soon things were beginning to happen to the strong, husky college boys . . . by about 4 p.m. that left two of ten hikers.

Naturally only great-grandfather Bragg made it all the way. Bragg is filled with stories like that. How I'd like not to be the one who conks out. Too little pride, I guess, or no previous respect for physical endurance. Now I wish for it. He's a man to follow.

I don't have to be sick at all, or get heart disease, I have been suffering pain when coming up the stairs and that's really scary. If 10 percent overweight you cut 20 percent off life, — 20 percent overweight, 40 percent off life expectancy. I am 25 percent overweight. According to this I died yesterday. And it's been close. I have felt that. I am going to memorize page 65 of Bragg.

Keep Your Morale High

I want you to understand that even when you take the one day fast, you are cleansing and purifying your whole body. The very thought that you are building a painless, tireless, ageless body should be an incentive to keep your morale high during your fast. Don't allow self-pity, or any negative thoughts, to get in your mind during your fast. Repeat these powerful affirmations all during the day you are fasting:

1. I have this day put my body in the hands of God and Nature. I have turned to the highest power for internal purification and rejuvenation.
2. Every minute that I am fasting, I am flushing dangerous poisons out of my wonderful body that could do great damage. Every hour that I am fasting, I am happier and happier.
3. Hour by hour my body is purifying itself.
4. In fasting, I am using the same method for physical, mental and spiritual purification that

the greatest spiritual leaders have used through-
out the ages.

    5. I am in complete control of my body dur-
ing this fast. No false hunger-pains are going to
make me stop fasting. I will carry my fast through
to a successful conclusion, because I will have
absolute faith in God and Nature.

    Just remember you must direct instructions
to the cells of your body with your subconscious
mind. Whatever thought you send to your body
is going to be carried out by your cells. . . .

                    — Paul Bragg, *ibid.*

I'm going to memorize it so I'll be tempted to use it.
This is the stuff which I've put down all my arrogant
intellectual life. I wasn't even ever disturbed by the fact
that the people who believed it all seemed very happy.
Misguided softheads. And see where my wisdom has got
me. You don't catch little fat Karen believing anything
that might help her. After all, it's surely better to be fat,
ugly, miserable, unloving, unloved, and unworthy than
to admit a wrong idea into one's pure lode.

Onward to the fasting path.

It's 1:30 and I'm hungry.

It's 2:30 and I'm happy. It's incredible how my body
reacts to half a day of fast. My mind is busy seducing
men in its suddenly recaptured bikini figure. I'll drop in
on Sydney and he'll see my long hair but will never know
about the 40 pounds I've gained since we stopped being
lovers and I replaced him with a cotton-candy machine.

I have a hunger pain which is strong enough to have
to be resisted. I resist and ten minutes later feel physical
and psychical energy. Everything is always psychological,
but isn't it possible that when the hunger didn't get fed
my body produced exactly what it needed — therefore
my surge of well-being?

Still first day. I fantasize giving other people advice on how to lose weight.

— Are you on a diet?

— Well, it's a permanent thing. (I speak with ease and the assurance a well-dressed, well-built woman always has.) It's what I don't eat mainly. I just don't eat anything that isn't natural. Or rarely. An occasional bit of cheese and butter, bread. Occasionally.

It is 5 o'clock. Think I can't make it. Hungry and depressed. Want to eat everything I saw on TV. How stupid of me to think I could watch TV and make it.

I'd like to eat an orange.

Oh, come on, Karen, you can make it through. Think about looking good at the Seder next week. Think of men. If you eat an orange and two eggs and cheese, that's 310 calories and you'll only lose a pound. Why go through all this and quit at 5? If you have to go to school tomorrow take an Ayds. And cross your fingers.

You won't be hungry after the third day, they all say. Tuesday, Wednesday, Thursday.

7 p.m. I didn't make it. 2 oranges, cheese soufflé. Now I want to go and buy German chocolate cake.

8:30 p.m. Out to have a binge. Did a certain sequence of events overcome me? Need to go to work. Did oranges and soufflé create a demand?

I am so tired of thinking about it. I botched it up again and am rushing writing this so I can eat my cake and ice cream.

After: I have done this awful thing again. Damn. I feel like never again, but oh, Jesus, I've felt like this before. Ready to go on a diet. I must not stay in bed. I'm wrong that I can run my life successfully from bed.

(53)

People's minds wander away from you as you talk.

I think it's look away, then listen away. Of course, maybe you've turned into a bore — but it's the same people who used to listen to you — and look at you.

A Black friend once explained to me that in a movie with Harry Belafonte and Sidney Poitier the reason the audience laughed when the Black woman walked right into the bank in full daylight and set things up and was stopped by no one, even though there were dozens of cowboys and bank people about, was that nobody sees Black people. I didn't know whether she really meant it, but it sure had broken up the audience, mostly Black. I think that's the way it is with fat women.

It is true that in a store no one sees me any more. At meetings I used to be called on pretty fast if I wanted to be. Now I rarely get recognized. All in my mind? I really doubt it.

(54)

Day one of still another fast: Fasting weight 185. There must be an incentive, I think. Different things will work at different times. The last time it worked for five days was at New Year's. Probably due to the natural impetus toward self-renewal which that always brings. I lost 10 pounds in five days....

Today the impetus is my editor's impending arrival. I've a headache, stomach ache, and heavy fatigue. Maybe all psychological. Maybe flu. At any rate, I'm here in bed. This time I'm trying liquids only, but including cocoa. A fattening but encouraging drink. I must keep in mind that within two days I will feel great.

Still day one of this fast: I've been in bed all day, aches, pains, general despondency. Ready to go off diet to feel better but am so depressed feel even eating won't help. Intense pain and aches and depression by 5 p.m. Started eating, beef dip and slaw, fritter, ice cream.

Want spaghetti again. In my family spaghetti is soul

food. The word is etching itself into my brain. If I do not get up, get dressed, and go out there and get it, surely earthquakes will burst upon the land. Tidal waves will reach Nebraska, if I do not get up and get spaghetti and eat it, nobly sacrificing myself for the greater glory of mankind. Also garlic bread and Coca Cola.

Didn't make it through the night. What good does writing this do me? There are no insights that heal. Just ones that hurt. I feel like I'm walking around inside a nervous breakdown. If I stop eating, will all of me split into pieces? There'd be heavy caloric pieces in the alleys tonight?

(55)

April already.

Pap smear. New doctor, no lecture on weight then. I slide the pound bar back. But we have both seen it, and the nurse too, at 187. I leave the bar at the 150, though. That's the least of it. Get my joke? Least. 187. So I came home and binged. I guess I ate so much that I felt the possibility of enough well-being to go on a fast.

It seems the only way that I can feel energy in me is by eating obsessively to the point of no more space anywhere, or by fasting. Why not fast forever then? This is where the psychology comes in.

I am ready to quit. I don't know where to go to turn in my fork.

(56)

I can't fast. Not even ten minutes any more. Strike that rush cure.

(57)

I am saved by Shelley Winters. I have loved her since The Poseidon Adventure. When she swam across that water, and permitted those underwater shots — wow — she helped all of us who would've let everyone drown, including ourselves, before showing off the braces in our undercoatings. And she has my disease. And used to be thin and beautiful and married to an actor who was thin and beautiful. She hasn't let the illness stop her. Tonight, again, there she is, her own woman. So good at what she does that you'd think she'd chosen that mode of living out of her own free will. I doubt that. I'll try again. That must be better than crying, I'd think. Except I never cry. Just bitch.

Thank God for the temporary cures. Without them your soul could not survive. Unalleviated self-disgust cannot last indefinitely. You will die in your deepest places even before you have made the final weight gain of the coffin.

(58)

A milk shake is soothing, though. Like resting in someone's arms. I'd better try to meet somebody anyway. But if I felt bad with George and Steven 20 pounds ago, what now?

(59)

Note on weight-losing procedures: Do not weigh. Go down size by size with your clothes. Blouses that button down the middle are best. You can see them get closer every morning after a 900-calorie or less day. The "I" this morning is consistent to the "I" that went to bed last night. That is, "I" am still sober. After 10 pounds, what happens to me? How can I prevent its happening?

I am trying to learn something and I keep getting defeated. I spot pieces of myself, the warring elements. I'll be damned if, after six hundred years in analysis, I know why they war.

I am tired of being a battlefield. How do I send the troops to another country?

There is a monster who must lie there in wait for me to finish a logical dinner, so he can begin to thrash about and demand to fill *his* belly. He isn't in the conversations about food plans, isn't in the debates, the diet puddings planned. He doesn't talk at all. He just waits. He hears the conversations with you and you and he just waits.

Dear God, it's an *I Ching* night.

What should I do to get help on the diet question?

12 changing into 25 Stagnation into Innocence. With 6 in the first place. 12 Stagnation: Heaven is above, drawing farther and farther away, while the earth below sinks farther into the depths. The creative powers are not in relation. It is a time of standstill and decline. The Judgement: Standstill. Evil people do not further.

The perseverance of the superior man.

The great departs; the small approaches.

Heaven and earth are out of communion and all things are benumbed. What is above has no relation to what is below, and on earth confusion and disorder prevail. The dark power is within, the light power is without. Weakness is within, harshness without. Within are the inferior, and without are the superior. The way of inferior people is in ascent; the way of superior people is on the decline. But the superior people do not allow themselves to be turned from their principles. If the possibility of exerting influence is closed to them, they nevertheless remain faithful to their principles and withdraw into seclusion.

Jesus Christ. How does it do it? I hope the small is really approaching.

6 at the beginning doesn't mean a damn thing to me. Onward to Innocence.

25 Wu Wang — Innocence (The Unexpected)

When movement follows the law of heaven, man is innocent and without guile. His mind is natural and true, unshadowed by reflection of ulterior designs. [What hope for me? I am an ulterior design.] For wherever conscious purpose is to be seen, there the truth and innocence of nature have been lost. Nature that is not directed by the spirit is not true but degenerate nature. . . . The Judgment: Innocence. Supreme success. . . . If someone is not as he should be, he has misfortune, and it does not further him to undertake anything.

Man has received from heaven a nature innately good, to guide him in all his movements. By devotion to this divine spirit within himself, he attains an unsullied innocence that leads him to do right.

In the *I Ching* all is well. I am very tired of all this struggle and I wish I had the soul to make it all well with myself. I am fat and hopeless and see no way into, or out of, the situation. There is something I need to see that I do not see. In my stagnation, in my innocence. Does heaven really have lines for me? If so, when do I get to know them? Are these hips and breasts to define me forever? Will I learn to accept it? Is that what all this is about?

(60)

The treachery of one "I" to another never stops.

(61)

Atkins Schmatkins
Stillman, Schmillman
Grapefruit, shapefruit

Encounter Group

How the hell did I get here? I listen to everyone, that's how. At lunch Suzi says we should go and Joyce says go. They both agree. "So you won't meet Prince Charming. So you're fat. At least you won't eat for two hours, and with driving time that'll be almost six hours."

"What do I need to have everybody look at me for?"

Suzi says, "One minute you say no one looks at you, now that they'll all look. Look, I'm tiny and I need to meet someone. Come for my sake. Not just fat people are lonely."

Put it to me that way and you get me.

We drive to just outside of La Jolla. Beautiful setting at least, high up, in a large circular house. Sponsored by some one or other New-Fangled Life Style Facilitations Groups, Inc. There are two "facilitators." Which is a good thing because the first one is about 26 and weighs 40 pounds more than I do. And is my height. But he's a man. Men get away with a lot. The other one is handsome and has a beautiful body. He walks with that assured gait of a man who knows he's attractive to women. I hate to think that I think about them the way they think about us, but sometimes I do. Neat Levis. I'll watch him facilitate.

There are about fifteen in the group. It is quickly apparent that there is an "in" group and a "flux" group. I am a flux group for sure. People get in the center and speak. Standing up while the rest sit. Everybody looks like everybody else. That's the general level of my observations these days. There's fat, and there's everybody else. I suspect something is getting wronger and wronger with my thinking.

They all say they're suffering. Except those who say

they're "in a good place right now." They did suffer, though, and they tell you so.

I am slightly panicky over a woman next to me. She is telling us that she may commit suicide. Her life sounds awful. Depression upon depression, crazy action upon crazy action. Can the group help her? Her son's on junk. She cannot go on. The group is warm but not upset. They appear to offer strength but they also want to know how with all the strength they offer she could still want to commit suicide.

Hey, fellows, her kid's in an alley shooting up.

They go on about the circle.

A lot of people here tonight evidently had planned to be at a retreat run by Clifford in a mountain place nearby. Cancelled at last minute. Each tells of his reactions to not seeing so and so at the retreat, but lots of the so-and-so's are here, and on *ad infinitum*. A scene of incest runs through the group — where did you find this one, Suzi?

The thing is we hunt and we think we find and. . .

My turn. On my feet, in the center of the group.

Warmly, professionally, kindly, my assholed Levi leader asks: "Karen, why are you angry?"

"I'm not angry."

"Yeah, you are angry."

"Why do you say that?"

"You don't like being fat. You want to take it out on me, the group."

Amazing. I was getting angry.

"Now, why are you so fat?"

I've had it. I'm going to start telling them.

"So I can be a foil for rotten cruel people like yourself."

"How can you say that to us? I only asked so we can help."

"You couldn't figure out an answer without having to ask the questions?"

"I wanted to involve your feelings. Your fat tends to isolate you."

"You have succeeded in involving my feelings. My feeling is that you are a shithead."

He says, "You're going to feel a lot better for saying that, you'll see." And I am allowed to sit down.

I sulk but I keep listening. What else can I do? Two guys are already tripping out over Suzi and that at least is nice. One of us will return to work Monday somewhat better off. And there are the six hours I'm not eating.

But something happens. Mid-group a lady opens the door and walks in. I immediately like her. She is middle-aged; her long gray hair is worn up, casually but femininely. She looks like she's brought up three children with competence and generosity. The people, the facilitators, know her, they smile, and she fits into the circle. She looks at peace. I'd like to be at peace. She isn't skinny, but she is thin enough. She's dressed comfortably. It's obvious those there who know her like her. Wonder what she'll have to say?

Her turn comes. The same facilitator who ripped at me asks her warmly, "Susan, how are you tonight?"

"Good, Bob," she says. "Cliff's in the hills leading the retreat so I thought I'd come over and say hello."

My first thought is, wow, married to a psychologist — she's together. But then the pieces of what others have said come together in my head. In another girl's head too.

"There is no retreat in the hills."

She is nice, Clifford's wife. There is no put down in her voice. "But there is, my husband is there right now."

Now there are a few who begin to see it. A man, settling it, says, "No, there's no retreat in the hills. It was cancelled this afternoon. The girl's right. I was to go too."

Jesus. Nobody says anything. Oh, my poor lady. You didn't even get fat. Just a little older than you had been.

After a minute the facilitator says, "Well, let's go on a bit, and then come back." His smile is that of a small boy not quite comprehending all the rules of the very game he's struggling to learn to play.

The lady bursts into tears and leaves.

The evening ends. On the way home Suzi tells me that the lady who is about to commit suicide is about to commit suicide every Saturday night meeting. Tells the same story too. One of the guys told Suzi this at the break.

"So we don't have to worry about her, Karen."

"No, I wasn't."

"Wouldn't it be great to be married to a facilitator?"

"Yeah."

It is three in the morning when I get home, but I eat. Why not? It's guaranteed to be there whenever you want it.

(63)

That encounter has triggered more than a binge. Questions in the head.

— Let's get to the nitty-gritty of this, Karen. If you weren't a compulsive overeater, how did you get to be one?

— Birth control pill?

— Oh, God, you dumb thing.

— Okay. Sydney may have had a lot to do with it. Oh, that I should have been ruined and fattened by a man with a name like Sydney. Just thinking about this, just talking about him, makes the hate come back. I'd like to dedicate a book to him: "Dear S. In hope of length of agony and continual groaning."

And I'll bet that at this moment, while I crave for a hatchet and a hot dog, he is no doubt having an orgasm. With a different girl at all his acupuncture points.

To believe that he, as well as I, draws energy within this cosmos, and in his place belongs to the universe, is for me to heal. I can usually do it for about ten seconds.

He'll reincarnate a viper.

I loved Sydney very much. I'll be a simpleton through eternity. I'm sure Kahlil Gibran could make something neat of all this hate. Couple it with love, no doubt, and announce it for a theory of the universe.

There is no one thirty-eight who has not been left by a lover.

(64)

I thought I was cured of the thought of Sydney, that I had eaten him to death. But they're both still here — the food and the thinking of.

So what if it began beautifully, on hot summer sand, the feeling, the statement that at last you'd found each other. Is it because I believed it and surely hadn't any longer been believing it with my recent lovers? Falling in love was turning into a posture, more than a state. With Sydney I believed it. Perhaps because he believed it — that may have been its charm. He explained it so well: until we'd met he'd never seen things at eye level. He'd never looked right at the reality of things.

Fuck, fuck, fuck, Mexico, Carmel, Alaska, would you believe? A year.

A trip on my own. Colorado Book Fair, hardly a desertion of one I loved. Returning to the first of the true confessions of how sorry he was he'd screwed around, but how a man needs his freedom. That's when you get off, girls, if you've a brain. I believed him. After all, he said it wouldn't happen again. God, was he sorry it had happened!

Now, lots of men play around. And the ideal playmate knows that the only way to truly love is to give freedom to the loved one. Hail to thee, Rollo May and Erich Fromm, both players, no doubt. And to the women coming up through women's lib who also seem to be able to play it that way, and to anyone who can play it that way.

But just let me tell him, at the right moment next time, before any hot beaches, shellfinding days, and purifying pledges, that I am not one of those new people. I'll say something witty like: well, if you're planning to hurt me, let's skip it, because if you do, I'll become a compulsive eater. Well, maybe not that.

He has a Mercedes, the expensive one. It's probably the only real love he's ever felt. Could I assign my kids at school to paint bunnies all over his car? Of course not, girls. There's nothing you can do but suffer.

Okay, but why remember any of it? Yet, certain days, it doesn't end. I remember the especially good times, the tenderness given and received. But then, as I'm softening in my image of him, the truth — the tenderness was given but not received. I received technique, the lie hidden by the liar. It is not like a marriage breaking up. (That was far easier; Jack and I ended something we'd begun together and been through together until it ended.) It is as though you've been made by an imposter. And once you know that, there's no way for your pain ever to lessen. He was never there at all. Only his shadow!

That's chocolate pudding there in the pot! Stir slowly. Use eye-level tablespoon.

It is humiliating to say that during our time he bought a house and obviously had no plans for me in it, and I still believed that he needed to complete his "maturation project," as he called it. He did, really, say that. He needed to mature slowly but he could not imagine a future without me. Christ, he must have had a 28-year mortgage. They could mature together. The pain is only half that he was such a vicious rotten bastard — three-fourths is that I believed him. I told that year's analyst that the house was only big enough for one person really. My analyst said, "That's preposterous. There's no house that is only big enough for one."

"Yes, there is. But soon [after the 28-year mortgage] we'll live together."

"Who says?"

"He does. I know that he loves me."

"Let's discuss your dreams."

"Banana splits," I said.

It's the fact that you were a fool that stays with you longest. There was another man I loved. But he never lied to me. I should've gotten out before I did, but at least he wasn't secretly making fun of me, sport of my body, putting poems into my pen.

There is the image of Sydney marveling at my colossal, omnipresent innocence.

Over and over.

Damn.

But, girls, there's always that question, isn't there? If with the paid-off mortgage he should come whistling at me, would I not go after him? Knowing then, that he had always loved me and would be with me finally?

Romantic, colossal, omnipresent innocence.

Him, me, and the mortgage. Joint coffins.

No, I wouldn't go with the cruel, evil person.

I'd rather eat!

(65)

I like to think of destroying his Mercedes. Marring it by contrasting signs: "McDonald's welcomes you," on each front fender, "Winchells is where I'm heading," on the rear fenders, and so on.

Sometimes I think only the ludicrous image can save me. But why do I have to become that image?

Everything lurks in all of us.

(66)

A good day. No binge. Calm from somewhere. Brought in by a breeze from offshore for all I know.

What one really wants to do is buy time. Buy when one is aware and alert and functioning and learn to let go of when one is not.

(67)

Ram Dass and Sattvic

> In India, foods are divided into three categories, which are called Tamasic, Rajasic, and Sattvic, and since the Hindu system is based on concern with consciousness we can listen to it with a certain kind of thoughtfulness . . . the Sattvic force is that which is toward consciousness . . . And it is suggested that when you are working on consciousness you eat primarily Sattvic foods . . . which turn out to be primarily limiting oneself to fruits, honey, nuts, dairy products . . . I don't eat meat, fish, chicken or eggs. I don't eat them because I am in a situation where I meet people in India who know how it is and they say, "Look, we don't eat them," and so I don't eat them because I'm a copycat because I want what they've got. That's the reason I don't eat them. I can't give you a very hip, sophisticated, rational model.

That's what I want — a hip, sophisticated, rational model, that by following will cure me of this obsession. I'll try Sattvic foods. Sattvic me from now on.

Purchased at health food store: 1. carrot juice, 2. corn, 3. squash Italian, 4. banana squash, 5. asparagus, 6. yogurt strawberry pushups, 7. ice cream, 8. three healthy candy bars (220 calories each, though one is lo-cal — only 175 calories), 9. carrot cake. Thank God for Sattvic.

I ate it all when I got home.

(68)

Now I want to eat the cantaloupe. And a Triscuit.

Voice: Who are you who helps me?

Voice: You know you can't. The first indulgence contains in it the final binge.

I: Who are you who helps me?

V: Your good self. Shall I call myself your Junior Size self?

I: But you seem masculine.

V: Well, a man wants a thin girl.

I: Has it been you all the time on my side?

V: Kid, you've had lots of help. Not enough, evidently.

(69)

"Joyce, I can't give the speech tonight."

"Why not?"

"I have nothing to wear."

"Call up the superintendent of our district and tell her to cancel the conference because you have nothing to wear."

"I'm not going to go."

"You have to go. Ben's coming. And if my husband is going to an education event, you can't cancel the event."

"Why is he coming?"

"To give me support to support you."

"You win. Good-bye. I'm off to Lane Bryant's." ("And here she comes, our California Sweetheart of the Week. What size today? Up, up and outward.")

I did it: "How to Teach Reading After the Damage Is Done." Audience seemed to like it.

Hope I was a credit to my disease.

(70)

I wake, feeling successful. I didn't come home and binge last night. And at dinner with Joyce at the Golden Temple Conscious Cookery, I remained conscious for the first time in ages. I ordered a salad and yogurt, and left some. Then I slipped a little and ordered dessert. I wanted Joyce to have cheesecake. Bullshit, I wanted to have cheesecake. The exciting thing was that I ordered this crazy thing called "wha pudding." When it came I didn't like it, so I didn't eat it. What a sense of power one can get over not finishing something. Most often I eat it regardless of whether I like it or not.

What ends a binge? Begins it? A time comes when I see myself clearly as killing myself. I eat until I pass out. The next day the binge is over. Has it been some form of religious sacrifice? Have I offered up my life and had it given back to me? I always feel born anew — now I can start dieting. Is it all just a psychological nuance of masochism? There, I've suffered enough, now I can start over.

It is no small pity, and should cause us no little shame, that, through our own fault, we do not understand ourselves, or know who we are. Would it not be a sign of great ignorance, my daughters, if a person were asked who he was, and could not say, and had no idea who his father or his mother was, or from what country he came? Though that is great stupidity, our own is incomparably greater if we make no attempt to discover what we are, and only know that we are living in these bodies, and have a vague idea, because we have heard it and because our Faith tells us so, that we possess souls. As to what good qualities there may be in our souls, or Who dwells within them, or how precious they are — those are things which we seldom consider and so we trouble little about carefully preserving the soul's beauty. All our interest is centered in the rough setting of the diamond, and in the outer wall of the castle — that is to say, in these bodies of ours.

— St. Theresa of Avila

(71)

Off to the Big Orthomolecular Psychiatrist

I have read at least ten books on hypoglycemia. The thing about that little disease is that it explains every symptom I've ever had in my life, from depression to headache.

Do I have it? My internist says no, but, damn, those books sure sound like me.

Scene. Peach office with trimmings of rosewood. $50.00 an hour.

I explain about the eating.

"Well, yes, let me give you these tests, get the record of your glucose tolerance test, and see you in a few weeks when I've got the results. Wash your hair and in three days send a batch of hair to this address."

I do as told and return. Eight pounds heavier. He doesn't seem to notice.

"You have hypoglycemia and the following vitamin and mineral deficiencies."

"My doctor says I don't have hypoglycemia."

"Most doctors don't know what's going on nutritionally."

"Does it have anything to do with my compulsive eating?"

"It could have, a little. We'll try you on the diet and see how you do."

"But I can't stay on a diet. I keep eating."

"Well, then I can't help you."

"Well, I'll try. Does it explain my extraordinary afternoon fatigue?"

"That it does, and if you get to the right food, that will go away. Plus take these vitamins." (Which can be purchased for three thousand dollars in the pharmacy downstairs.)

"What can I do about the compulsive eating?" (I am on the verge of tears, which is rare with me. But where do I turn now? He's supposed to be the most helpful person. He's been so highly recommended that surely he can do something.)

"Stop eating so much."

I smile wanly. "That seems to be my problem, doctor."

Laughing, he says, "Don't worry. If worse comes to worst, you can always have your jaws bolted together. That seems effective."

The dumb bastard is pleased. He continues chuckling.

"I don't think that's funny, Dr. Ortho."

"Oh, why not?"

"Well, maybe if you were sitting on this side of the desk and looked the way I look, maybe then you would see why it isn't funny."

"Ah, I see."

"Good-by, Dr. Ortho."

At home later. What difference does it make what you have? Hypoglycemia or not. The trick, baby girl, is you'll never know why about anything. Stop living in the problem, start living in the solution.

Where's the solution?

In the same place in which it would be if you have hypoglycemia. Stop eating sugar. Sure, something is physically different with you.

People who can stop eating do stop eating.

I try to fall asleep wondering what Dr. Ortho'd say to his mother if she were having her leg amputated from diabetes. Make that his leg. I'm angry and I grow meaner. Both legs.

(72)

I am finding myself spending more time with heavier people. Cultivating those with like problems. Had dinner with X and then went to see the movie *Cry the Beloved Country*. Elegant little restaurant, food delicate and delicious. Try this, try that. God knows if we even talked to one another. Then, I had picked the theater carefully on a mall with B & R. I took half of the freezers into the theater with me.

I was thinking in the movie that art is made by the people of many selves, not by the single-minded or single-hearted. Of course that's probably not true — just if I'm ever to create something of art, it had better be true at least for me.

May 20.

Starting again. Even one day off the streets now is a blessing. And inexplicable. A gift.

(73)

Five days later.

Jubilance ended today, suddenly, after school. Since then I have eaten: peanut butter and jam, three large Mrs. Good's, chicken and French fries, strawberries and whipped cream, ice cream, vanilla, ½ pint, and ice cream, chocolate, ½ pint, spaghetti.

I am Lon Chaney, Jr., turning into the werewolf. It comes upon me, and it takes over.

56

(74)

May 20, '75

Marilyn sent me an article by Dr. B on his work with
depressed patients in a mental hospital. It sounds good.
She circled where it says in the notes that he also does
well with obesity patients. He's far away, but I am so
desperate. Why not?

May 24

After putting it off with four days of bingeing and what
would I say to him anyhow that I haven't already said
to others, I finally made the appointment. $75.00 an hour.
Why not? Same desperation today as every day. Hope,
at any price, would be cheap. I'll have to drive to Ojai
to see him. But at least he'll see me soon: I'll go.

May 30 (To be known in my head henceforth as Behav-
iorist Massacre Day)

The first thing wrong was with the road to Ojai. It
does not have the usual accouterments of binge places.
Fortunately I had started the drive with three ice-cream
sandwiches (the maximum that can be eaten before the
last one melts through its paper and onto your dashboard
to form eternal rivulets of hardened calories) and a pound
of caramels. Not having places to stop, I arrived early
for the appointment. Found a place with shakes. Quite
near the office, I noted. I wondered if he could just find
a nice place for me in the hospital if I told him how
my thinking and action had gone on this nice quiet day's
drive to Ojai.

I went in willing.

He was tall and skinny; very homely, but bearded, one
of those men who have taken a lot of trouble to make
themselves look as well as they can. He wasn't fatherly
— when I was a kid the doctor sat on the bed and held
my hand and I've been looking for the same man ever
since — but he was skinny. A very good sign.

Dr. B: I see your problem of course. What else?

K: Depression.

Dr. B: Look, if I stopped you on the street and I said, what things are bugging you, in order, what would you say?

K: Compulsive overeating, too much sleeping, which is the depression. I liked where you said in your article that overeating is a depressive equivalent. That sort of made sense to me.

Dr. B: Other problems?

K: I can't stop eating.

Dr. B: What else have you tried? To stop eating?

K: Not a lot too extensively. I tried diet pills for four days a year or so back. And at the end of the four days, I was a nervous wreck, my head going through ceilings, and I could binge completely right over the pills. This should stop me from eating, I'd think, and go right on.

Dr. B: What else? Usually there's everything.

K: I went to a meeting of OA once but it's too religious for me.

Dr. B: OA is better than almost anything else. But it's a drag.

K: Yeah. You know pills attract me more and more, though. To keep me awake. But I'm afraid of pills.

Dr. B: You won't need pills. My method works.

K: Eating has destroyed me. I mean, you know, I've never had a problem like this. There's nothing. It's incredible.

Dr. B: Religion?

K: Jewish, but with some Christianity, Hinduism, Buddhism, and a few other isms thrown in. Altered states of consciousness loom as a coming religion.

Dr. B: No fat Hindus.

K: Buddha was fat.

Dr. B: He wouldn't have been if he'd seen me.

Damn. I make myself angry. I was already getting clues that I didn't like this man. But he was the doctor. I kept laughing at his little witticisms. Nothing was funny, but I'm always sociable. (Isn't that pretty blood I have, flowing out there in the street, I'd probably say at a car accident, if somebody asked me in a nice tone of voice what I thought of all that gushing.)

Dr. B: How many children?

K: None.

Dr. B: Marriages?

K: One. Over by 20.

Dr. B: Present living circumstances?

K: Myself and two animals. (He wrote down the names of the animals.)

Dr. B: Education, any advanced degree?

K: One and three-fourths Masters.

Dr. B: In?

K: Elementary Education with a Reading Specialization. Three-fourths in English Lit.

Dr. B: Why only three-fourths?

K: I stopped caring what Beowulf said to Gilgamesh.

Dr. B: Boyfriends, sex life?

K: None, now.

Dr. B: How do you feel about that?

K: Well, a friend that I hadn't seen for a while asked me the other night how I'd been and I said, "I'm not going to talk about it, things have been too bad," and she said, "Well just give me two sentences," and I'll tell you the two sentences that came into my head.

Dr. B: What were they?

K: One was, nobody loves me, which I could have said, and the other was, I'm a compulsive overeater, which I couldn't get out of my mouth.

Dr. B: How are you physically?

K: Okay. One doctor says hypoglycemia, another doesn't.

Dr. B: Hypoglycemia is depression.

K: That's what my internist says.

Dr. B: Do you itch or sigh more frequently?

K: Do I what?

He repeated it. (Something I'd never thought about at all. See, they do know things we don't know.)

K: Sigh.

Dr. B: So far you've itched, but not sighed.

K: Oh.

He wrote that down too. (His pad now must have read: Annie, Hepburn, she itches.)

Dr. B: How'd you get a jaw line like that?

K: What?

Dr. B: Too much determination. You work too hard.

K: No, I don't.

He got out a mirror and showed me my jaw as though something was wrong with it. His showing me my jaw line was suddenly as painful as the stirrups, but at least you know what they're looking for there.

Dr. B: Look at this joint measure from here to here. Not stubborn enough. But determined. Think about the difference, for they are different. You're grim. Grim just doesn't make it.

K: I'm grim?

Dr. B: Yep. I've seen lots of little ladies like you, and most of them are possessing enormous quantities of anger and basically they are depressed because they're pissed to a fare-thee-well and no one will pay any attention to them. They are totally ineffective to whip the world into shape, depressed over ineffectiveness of anger, rather than a *per se* depression. For example, I don't detect any lack of feelings of personal worth. I mean, you don't have a great self-image but that's related to your weight and decreased self-functioning and that's not relative to you as a person. Is that right?

K: Well, I. . .

Dr. B: I mean, you don't dislike yourself.

K: Well, everyone's been telling me I'm very negative.

Dr. B: How do you feel about yourself?

K: Very negative.

Dr. B: Eliminate the eating — outside of that are you all right?

K: There is no outside of that anymore. That's why I'm here. And it's not the being fat. It's the eating I'm doing.

Dr. B: Well, then onward to my theory, which you mustn't steal, although you need my charisma to make it work.

At last his theory. God forbid I should steal it. It, elaborately, amounts to picking up less food with your fork eventually. Tricky. Behavioral junk.

K: Uh, I've tried to tell you this a lot of times, but I don't think you're listening to me. As bad as the weight is, it's the eating that's worse.

Dr. B: Don't worry about the eating. It's fun.

K: It's fun?

Dr. B: Obviously, look, if you're eating that way, it's fun. Look, here's the girl, here's the food, and they are making a mush of each other. Now I will say it again and maybe it will get into your head. If you're eating, it's what you want to do. It ruins the word "compulsive" completely. Get rid of that word. You should always beware of words that don't have a referent. Compulsive doesn't have a referent.

K: It does to me.

Dr. B: No, it doesn't. Compulsive sounds as if it explains something but it doesn't. Human beings can't bend a finger unless they want to. You can't be forced to do anything. You decide to do something, whatever you do is basically what you want to do. Regardless of what you say about it, no species of life can do anything except what it wants to.

K: You look back and think I did what I wanted to do?

Dr. B: Yes. Definitely.

K: What about complexes?

Dr. B: I don't use those words. Those are labels, myths.

K: Look, when I've been sitting there, after bingeing for several days. . .

Dr. B: Don't use obese talk. We'll just be using skinny talk.

K: Look, I'm sitting there, putting those chocolates into my mouth.

Dr. B: They're good, aren't they?

K: No, listen to me.

Dr. B: Are they yummy?

K: No.

Dr. B: Yes.

K: No. (I am practically frantic. He doesn't hear me.)

Dr. B: If they tasted like moths, would you eat them?

K: Look, that's what I'm trying to tell you. I'm praying, let me stop, let me stop, and I keep eating.

Dr. B: That's called mind fucking and you might as well give it up.

K: Yeah, it's mind fucking. Especially when I'm sitting here overpowered by your personality.

Dr. B: Right, well, you'll use my personality to get skinny. Now, let's get back to my process. (His process, as he calls it, includes eating as much as you want and watching people eat. Oh Christ, he's an amateur. He should be an adjunct of Weight Watchers, next to the scale, on again, off again.) Don't finish all of everything.

He thinks that's original. *Woman's Day, Ladies' Home Journal,* and the L.A. *Times* publish it daily: "How to Cut Your Food in Small Pieces and Cut Your Weight in Half."

K: You mean I can have a gallon of ice cream but leave a little bit?

Dr. B: Right.

K: I think I can handle that. (If it's Neapolitan, what flavor do I leave a little bit of?)

Dr. B: You can have all you want to eat and still lose.

K: But how do I get to want to do it?

Dr. B: I don't give a fuck. You don't need to do it. You want to stay fat, that's okay. You want to stay that way. Your upper lip's too skinny.

K: My upper lip's too skinny?

Dr. B: It doesn't matter if you want to stay chubby. You have to find the carrot, that's your job, maybe it's hospitals and needles, pussy falls out, bypass. You find the carrot. And if you don't do what I say, it's because you're angry. You know, if I tell this whole thing to twelve people, one listens.

K: Is that right?

Dr. B: One loses weight immediately, rapidly, pleasantly, no paranoia.

K: What of the eleven left?

Dr. B: I don't give a fuck about them. Why should I? I helped one out of twelve.

K: Okay. Now let's take another one of the twelve and say it didn't work and the reason it didn't work was her anger, what should she do?

Dr. B: Learn to do what she's told.

K: What if she can't?

Dr. B: She needs education. Which she gets here.

K: But you said you only see people a few times.

Dr. B: True, you can't fuck around. Complying at one level, but not on another.

K (I swoop. Can I get him to answer anything for me?): Levels, that's complex, you know. How to change levels? That's the problem.

Dr. B: No. You only have one problem. Don't tell me this is difficult. You'll get skinny, lose depression, or keep it, or any alternative. You choose. Be my guest. Do you follow me? If you don't stop eating, you don't want to.

K: Look, you don't have the problem.

Dr. B (jumped up and screamed at me): I weighed two hundred and fifteen and there was no program. I had to make it up.

K: Look, when you wanted to stop eating. . .

Dr. B: I didn't want to stop eating.

K: When you wanted to be skinny, when you consciously wanted to stop. . .

Dr. B: You don't stop eating with this program.

K: You're not hearing me.

Dr. B: Look at your jaw line. Just look at your jaw line.

K: My jaw line?

Dr. B: Are you willing to give up?

K: Give up what?

Dr. B: Running your own life.

K: That's what they want in OA. To whom?

Dr. B: To me. Temporarily I'll be your green man in your head. Just don't trust your own brain; you'll have to trick yourself into doing anything good. You think you're trying to get out of depression but you're choosing to stay where you are. You think things should be as you see it. Not at a conscious level.

K: A few minutes ago, we didn't have an unconscious level.

Dr. B: I'm talking about inside the head. How it works.

K: Well, I am too.

He went on, repeating himself. Until we made another appointment. And I know I thanked him when I left.

If only all of me could have been angry. But deep down I always think everybody else is right. I found a supermarket and loaded up. So much for the ride to Ojai.

Wonder what happened to the other ten out of my twelve?

(75)

"Joyce, it is hopeless. I am hopeless."

"He just wasn't a nice person, Karen. Don't feel hopeless. It will change. You'll be all right, I know it."

Thank God for friends. Two minutes with Joyce should cost $75.00.

(76)

Complexes

June, nearly a school year gone.

I see something at last. It feels freeing to me.

The very worst thing about being this compulsive eater is not the qrotesque way I look. That's horrible enough. Far worse is acting the grotesque way I act. Next worst, is my constant condemnation of this way that I look and act.

Who hates me the most?

Compulsive eaters of the world, who hates you the very most?

I hate me the most.

You hate you the most.

No one could come closer to total hatred than we of ourselves. We are put down by everyone, but no harder put down than by ourselves. We listen and we listen to those damned outsiders and then, in our heads, we replay their conversations.

But I think I have made a discovery that will make us feel somewhat better about ourselves.

You know "I," right? The voice we think with, the voice we read with, the voice we talk to ourselves and to others with, this "I," the one from "I will go to the movies, I will study astronomy, I will go on a diet." This time "I" will stay on a diet. "I" will eat nothing at that party.

This "I," multitudinous as it is, for the "I" of astronomy is not necessarily the "I" of dieting, is not always the controlling factor of our actions. Now you say, Obviously, sometimes I do go out and eat a lot, even though "I" doesn't want to; I just can't seem to stop myself. I am a pig, I guess, just no self-discipline. I guess I'm hopeless.

No, Damn it, no. You, in any form you have ever had going in your head: you do not go out and binge. Something in you which is not "I" takes your body out on a binge and thus far in your life, you must go along. Then you eat, and then you next hear yourself getting two "I"s with voices: (1) Oh, that's good, and (2) I don't want to be doing this. And then the two voices go on until the binge ends. What ends this binge? You pass out.

What I am saying is that an unconscious complex remains unconscious. So? But, practically, what I am saying is that the complex forcing us to eat is nonverbal. We suppose all thinking or action must stem from verbal instructions. Kill Hilter, divorce Richard Burton, etc. But the eating complex does not act through a verbal nature. It is no less forceful therefore. In fact it is more forceful therefore. It controls me: while my mind talks to itself, the complex controls me, moves my legs, my mouth, my teeth, my memory and my speech; it can exert force and control me even while the complex I hear in my head at any given moment may be totally different.

In my head: No, I won't eat anything.

Action: Buys food.

In head: Please, God, let me throw it away. I don't want it, why can't I control it, of course I can, surely I can. Obviously all I need to do is not put it into my mouth. Physically I can control it. Is it because I broke up with whoever? Is it because I don't work diligently enough, is it because, is it because, is it because?

Action: Begins to eat food, proceeds until loss of consciousness.

Some people doubt there is an "I" at all. I don't believe this, though it's interesting for thinking about.

Is there any place for me to anchor? I think I can safely recognize as "I" the self that is constantly crying, I want to be thin. I want to have my body back. I don't. I don't want to be crazy. That self, that "I," cries right through our binges. We want to make that "I" the prevailing one.

Maybe that "I" in me is not my strongest "I," but it does want to choose life over death. Perhaps it's not my basic ego. Fuck jargon. My strongest "I" is out to kill me and won't even enter a dialogue. It doesn't need to speak to me to win battles. It comes with a nuclear warhead and feeds on ice cream and the etcetera.

So the trick is how to change your actions without any discussions of the issue.

Malaria is an action. Epilepsy is an action. Measles is an action. If you had any of these you would train yourself to feel physical symptoms that would be the clue that you were on the verge of illness, you would not condemn yourself for having the disease. You would take all the advice and medicine you could get and go on with your "I"s as best you could under the conditions of being sick. The physical engagement would be sufficient unto itself. You'd wait it out, praying possibly, but you'd be unlikely to want to kill yourself for being so rotten through and through that you had no self-discipline.

What do they say to us?

They say, Eat sensibly. Obviously you want to eat more than you want to be thin. When you want to be thin enough, you'll stop eating. If you'd just binge on carrots, it'd be okay. You're self-indulgent. And it's only a question of will power. Won't power, hah, hah, hah.

The complex possesses a body of its own. It just happens to be your body.

Your eating self has never heard of carrots. As to self-indulgent, if that's so, how come you don't have anything you really want?

Will power? Whose? I've got lots. But the beast within, underneath, Complex A, has got the body weight on his side.

I see that the only way to salvation is to be able to sense the power of the clues to the complex as it sneaks in on me. You need to have the reaction time of a Billie Jean King to be able to respond to something before it gets to you — if it gets to you, it's likely to be too late. It's quite a talent to be able to discern what may be coming at you even before it has begun its trip. It may be the job of a lifetime.

Somehow it helps me to think of the matter this way. It gives me a certain detachment I have not had before. Cancer is cancer and goes its own way. You have to treat it as best you can. But not by whip. Not by whip, any more.

(77)

Do a little something for your complexes every day.
    Sing a song of complexes
    All together in our solar plexus
    Why oh why will complex hex us?

    Sing a song of complexes.

    A penny for your complex.

(78)

A strong force to say "yes" to life falls upon certain writers. This is because so much inside them is of a deathly nature that they are arguing the issue of life and death daily. They hope that by putting it all "outside," they can, at least temporarily, find themselves inside the "yes." Most of mankind does not even know to be grateful for the "yes" they have inside them at all times.

(79)

To go wrong and not to alter one's course can definitely be defined as going wrong.

— Kung Fu meditation

Part Two

Respites and Surrender

Meditation means surrender, total letting go. As soon as someone surrenders himself he finds himself in the hands of divinity. If we cling to ourselves, we cannot be one with the almighty. When the waves disappear, they become the ocean itself.

— Bhagwan Shree Rajneesh

... You might say she tried to surrender something that she had not yet found.

— Reshad Feild

Question: What is that you call atman [soul]?
Answer: Really, no matter what we call it, we will miss it.

— Rajneesh, again

End of June
Creating My Imaginary Doctor.
I am reading *The Well Body Book*. I've really gotten
into health and nutrition. I wouldn't want to be killing
myself with sugar and not know the exact mechanism
by which the death was being brought about. I am reading,
and will try anything, everything. For today's reading,
we have "Creating My Imaginary Doctor":

> If you do not stop here to create your imaginary
> doctor you are passing up one of the most useful
> tools ... this character will become your alter
> ego, advisor, or helper ... The people of many
> cultures down through history, including some
> American Indians, created personal spiritual
> advisors to guide and assist them throughout life
> ... If when doing the exercise and getting an
> imaginary doctor, you feel that you are making
> the whole thing up (and perhaps you even feel
> a little bit silly), understand that these feelings
> are exactly right. Most people do feel this way
> at first. But once you have him or her, your imagi-
> nary doctor becomes a very useful tool, and in
> that way a reality.

See, I am willing to get to my imaginary doctor. What's
wrong with me? I can't find any literature or any doctor
here in the real world who agrees with anyone else.
  I am sitting in bed, yogi fashion. I am surrounded by
candy, ice cream dishes (empty), and a few more nutritious
binge foods like nuts and raisins ... I'm ready to find
a new doctor.

> The imaginary doctors might have objective reali-
> ties of their own; several people report having
> met their imaginary doctors in real life after creat-

ing them in the exercise. We found that the imaginary doctors act with their own personalities and idiosyncracies and not as though they were a part of your conscious mind . . .

I set myself to reach my imaginary doctor. First you breathe for a bit, so I breathed. Then, you imagine a house. I did; then the land, then the entrance. Finally, after much ado, you get to open the door and see your doctor.

I found myself in the desert, darkening desert, sun gone but light somehow present still in bits and pieces. Right away I wasn't sure I was in the right place. Who could have a practice there?

I went farther. There were bushes in the shape of mysterious animals, mysterious rocks in the shapes of birds, everything was losing and gaining first one reality and then another. I wondered where I was, and why I wasn't more frightened.

Part of me knew I was doing the thing and looking for my imaginary doctor. But part of me was in the desert looking sheepishly at every shape, wandering about on the rocks trying to discern the correct path I should take.

"Take the path with heart," I heard from that place where all that we have ever read and deeply felt in response to that reading takes place. Then I knew where I was, what country my meditation had brought me to, and who it was I was looking for.

I remembered the first time that Castaneda had gone to Don Juan. I was prepared if necessary to roll on the floor until I had found my spot. Perhaps the reason I had grown so heavy was that nowhere had I found my spot. Nor had I ever trusted or bled enough yet to roll over each inch of space until I might find myself. I read a lot.

"So," my fucking intellect said, "you've taken yourself

to Don Juan country. Castaneda addressed Cal Tech in a short haircut and Brooks Brothers sport shirt and already you're off in the desert."

But I kept walking, having by now forgotten all directions, but having accepted the visible reality before my eye. I awaited coyotes. But assumed I could count on some sorcerer or other to help me.

I tried to make light of my imagination. The experience was too powerful, too real, for me to deal with in any other way. For no money, for no thin body, for nothing, would I give up the certainty of a crowded McDonald's and the noise of a crowded schoolyard truly to find in some desert that there may be no need for anything except the spirit to play free and easy with the mind — and let the body do what it may. I want to be thin on the schoolyard. A man may have flown like a bird with a rock chained to its feet. That's fine and I'd pay heavy for a ticket, but on no account will I be that flier.

Which I do believe is what separates the true adventurers from the rest of us.

But since I was here I should look for the man I'd been sent for. Maybe it wouldn't be Don Juan but some apprentice. I might have an apprentice full-blown in my unconscious, but hardly a master union man.

I approached the house. The door opened and Don Juan came out to meet me. Every line of his face was not only Indian, wise, and obviously pure, but medical as well.

— You have come a long way here to have me for your doctor.

— Yes, will you be?

— Yes, I am. Tell me about you.

— Well, to begin with, you see, this fat I'm carrying.

— I do not see fat.

Was there a mirror around? I sure hadn't come all this way for Don Juan to have illusions about me.

— I'm very overweight and I can't stop eating.

— Peyote?

Offer or question?

— No, thank you. I don't care for any.

He looked at me with pity. I had found a caring doctor. So here I was on the desert and the prescription was for peyote to cure overweight. Chocolate peyote?

— Do you recommend anything else, sir?

— Yes.

He stepped toward me, I toward him.

— What?

He said three words. I didn't quite catch them. Or he had switched to some dialect I wouldn't even remember long enough to take back to my country to have translated.

— I didn't quite get that, sir.

He said the words again, and as he spoke he turned away from me and back toward his house. Before he reached his doorway, entered, and closed the door behind him, it had become dark and I was stranded in the desert.

"Don't eat sweets," he had said.

(1)

It is strange to me that at the same time that I am going on eating and eating, almost becoming acclimated to the totally destructive nature of my life, another kind of life, a strangely creative one, is increasing its grip on my awareness. Marilyn, deeper into more research stemming from her book *The Brain Revolution*, is drawing me further into the world of altered states of consciousness, God, and the Universe.

She says, with Joyce, and against a lot of evidence, that I'll stop eating eventually and that in the meantime I should try to stop suffering long enough to tune into the world about me. She is very convincing. Wants me to go to a weekend seminar led by Jack Schwarz. She swears he's something else again and I have been impressed by some of the things she's repeated that he has said.

I went to the Jack Schwarz seminar with Marilyn and I am so glad I did. Along with all the other astonishing things I felt today, in the Western Reserve and Trust Building amid the plush rugs and inner corridor trees lit by scattered skylights, I felt for the first time in a long time that I was near the doctor who had sat on the bed and held my hand when I was a kid.

I'm willing to bet that of the forty of us there I wasn't alone in my response to Jack. Intellectual content there was plenty, and spiritual guidance, but equally special was that as the day progressed, there was emotional presence also. We got friendly toward one another — all of us, old, young, thin, even a few fat people, some teenagers, all of us, by the first break, noticed one another and relaxed together.

Jack is tall, thin, a Westernstyle yogi, with a gray goatee and an intense look in his eyes. Within twenty minutes of listening to him I realized that I had already moved from one stage of consciousness to another. The first thing he said — and it was at these words that I felt a new vision encroaching upon my tired, used-up rational mind — was: "Everything is everywhere — all knowledge, all events. Think of it this way, if I turn on the radio right here I can get Los Angeles. If I turn on a stronger radio I can get Paris, any place in the world. But Paris, every place, it's here right now, isn't it?"

And onward from there. The seminar was seven hours, in the course of which he repeatedly shook all of my born-in-Brooklyn assumptions about the universe and reality.

A woman raised her hand to ask a question. She looked in the pink of health to me. Acknowledging her raised arm, he said, "That back pain needs low massage. I'm afraid you'll have it for a while." She looked shocked, having said not one word yet. He said, "I didn't read your mind. I see it in your aura." I wondered what he'd see in mine — carbohydrate layer one, carbohydrate layer two, how far down to get to me?

Toward the end of the time I saw him actually take a 6-inch-long needle, which he first dropped on the floor and stepped on. "So much for sterilization," he said. "Yes, there are germs all over, but I'm telling my body not to let them grow in me." Then he pushed the needle through his upper arm. In one hole and out the other. No blood. He talked blithely on through the whole thing. "I'm not really doing it, it's mass telepathy, they'll tell you."

Marilyn glanced at me. "Wow," her smile said. I sent an equally formidable "wow" back. I'd heard about it, but I doubted I'd ever really see it happen right in front of me. Jack showed us the holes in his arm, but within minutes they closed up.

"I didn't stick a needle through my arm," he said, "but through *an* arm." He said it was a matter of nonattaching himself to the idea of pain. We could all learn it.

I am not about to start with needles.

(3)

The only time I feel good lately is when I'm into reading this kind of stuff. Even the movies have begun to fail me since they mean running up and down the aisle for more food. Now, books can get me through a lot.

I never feel a greater security than in the first knowledge that a book is going to hold me all the way through. I don't always read it right away; that's like using up money in the bank. But in the back of my mind I know I have the greatest protection of myself in the world.

This consciousness stuff is already producing unique experiences in my life.

Yesterday I heard the words "Sai Baba" for the first time. Somehow it came up with Marilyn and it clicked.

All she said was something like, have you read about
Sai Baba, or maybe that some friend of hers had gone
to India to see him and had just returned and was spread-
ing the word around. I said, no, I hadn't heard of him,
and that was that.

Now tonight my friend Nor had to drop something
off here and came with her friend, Mary, whom I'd only
met once or twice before, never spoken to. I was reading,
off in biofeedback somewhere. I offered them coffee and
soon I was learning that Mary's daughter had just spent
a year in a monastery in India.

That's really a thing to hear, you know. The girl is
something like 24 and can go off to an ashram. If I'd
tried that, my parents would've said, "What do you need
an ashram for, you're pretty enough. You'll get a husband." Those of us women who just missed being liberated
have the urge to push the years back — not too many
would be necessary — and head for the ashrams and
the RNA molecules and mixed tennis tournaments.

"With whom?" I asked.

"Swami Sachitananda."

"He's one I don't know too well. Does he have a following in this country?"

"A small one."

"Did she like it?"

"Yes . . . now she's going to Sai Baba's for some months,
not sure how long."

There it was again, casually dropped. I almost always
refuse to believe in Jung's synchronicity as an explanation
for anything, but it does seem an odd coincidence.

"I've just begun hearing about him."

"I have the book with me. Do you want to borrow
it?"

"Yeah, I'd like to."

My mind has been thoroughly occupied with relatively

unobsessive thoughts for twenty minutes or so. But agonies will out:

"What does your daughter eat in the ashrams?"

(4)

Baba is written by the right person, Arnold Schulman. I can tell he grew up in my Brooklyn street school of "Don't believe anything that sounds out of the ordinary." I can trust him. If he spends a fortune to go to India to see if this guy he's been hearing about did or didn't materialize objects, cure people, and draw holy ash from empty air, I can trust his book.

I'm reading in it and it has an effect on me that is different from that of any book I've ever read. I'm reading it slowly. It's like Baba himself is drawing me in. I believe in the materializations and the other miracles. Naturally one of me is thinking it could all be good magic tricks, but I know Schulman has considered all of that and guarded against deception. I just plain find myself believing in it.

(5)

Today, still under the spell of the book and not bingeing terribly much I headed for the Bodhi Tree Book Store. Maybe there'd be something else about Baba. I passed a bulletin board and my eye caught: Sai Baba Center. A real center, near Santa Monica & Fairfax, not far from Canter's (old joke: if you want to open a pizza parlor, find a Jewish neighborhood). Where else would Sai Baba be? I went there.

New world. Records, films, tapes, chanting on Fridays, and movies of Baba several nights of the week. The first man I spoke to had been with Baba months before. I bought everything they had. Baba on Life and Death, photos of Baba, poster size, and all other sizes down to wallet size.

His photographs show a starkly intense and at the same time innocent face. He is a dark Indian, wears a long, orange robe and a bushy Afro-natural. His pictures glow. I've put them all over the house. Some devotees have had holy ash come forth out of the photographs. I haven't. Yet. Where I am living right now, through Baba, in this space, I believe that if I ever believed enough, ash would come out of the photograph.

I signed up for Chanting One — Introductory.

(5)

> ... the lesson that seemed to emerge for a person with my history of forgetfulness, doubts and hesitations was, as Hamlet put it so heartrendingly to himself: "the readiness is all." If one is truly ready within oneself and prepared to commit one's readiness without question to the deed that follows naturally on it, one finds life and circumstance surprisingly armed and ready at one's side ...
>
> — Laurens van der Post

May I have a pound of readiness please, with some cole slaw and potato salad on the side?

(6)

The center is an old house which has been turned into a worshiping place. You leave your shoes in the hallway.

Before I start to chant I look over the crowd. All of the men have beards. A few look as if the closeness to Fairfax Avenue has rubbed off onto their chanting and they move back and forth in a slow, hypnotic rhythm.

They are *dovining*. Rabbi Sai Baba. The women are in long dresses, almost saris, or they are in Levis. Indian shirts move back and forth in unison. There are no fat people in the room.

I turn my attention to the chanting. Of course I don't know the words — I never get the words of anything in another language (Hare Krishna chant took me about three years of constant exposure to on street corners to learn, and it only has six or so words in it. I had to get out of Nicheren Sho Shu: they have a litany!) I sort of murmur along with the group. But the people seem warm and gentle and are certainly enthusiastic. Baba's presence fills the room. There is an altar before me, with candles burning in front of a large picture of Baba. A drum accompanies the chanting and it all feels good. I think that if I asked Baba to help me lose thirty pounds, I could lose thirty pounds. Oh come on, Karen baby. Cut it out. Come on now.

But the trouble is I never believe enough. I am always cut off from the complete "readiness." Marianne Moore once said: "You are never truly free until you are made captive of supreme credulity." Why can't I just hang onto one thing for a while? Rest some place. Carrying this weight around is a lot of work. I seem to be carrying it from place to place. I'd be satisfied right now to leave it in any one place for a while.

After chanting, they showed a film. This Sai Baba is the reincarnation of the last Sai Baba. He is clearly a man expressing the largesse of his spirit. He says he will live until 96 and has already announced where his next incarnation will be. Bodies on, bodies off, with ease yet. He must be the man who could help me.

The director of the center speaks to me. A man who looks at peace with himself.

"Hello, did you enjoy the chanting?"

"Yes, thank you, I did."

"I remember you from when you bought all the material."

"Yes."

"I hope you'll continue coming. Baba does change one's life."

(I want to ask the man what he eats, but I can't just bring it up.)

"I was wondering, um-m-m, do you, does Baba, recommend any kind of food?"

"Less, I would say."

(Oh my God. How could he? But now he looks embarrassed.)

"I mean, less and less meat, aiming toward vegetarian."

"Oh, I see."

(8)

Chicken Conversation

— Baba, help me please. Appear in a dream.
— You don't need a dream. Eat fruit and nuts only for thirty days.
— What do I do with the chicken in the refrigerator?
— Throw it out.

Faith, and one can move mountains, declaim ash. I don't throw out the chicken and I know I won't eat fruit and nuts for thirty days.

(9)

But I'm not bingeing. It has been ten days now of going to the center and not bingeing. Eight pounds. The Sai Baba Diet and Chanting Production Company: can this be it?

(10)

Tonight at the center, in silent meditation, between the chanting and the films (God, he is beautiful, smiling, blessing, walking among his people, healing and giving), the obsession came over me. Everyone in the living-room chapel is praying quietly under his breath, or whispering a mantra, or deep in contemplation. Right up front, right in front of Baba's smiling, worshiped countenance, a banana split appears. No, I will not think of a banana split. I will think of an elephant instead.

Go away, banana split. Go to New Delhi. Please go away. The battle rages within me. I could just eat that one and then I could concentrate on the meditation again. Banana split switches to hot fudge sundae. They're chanting again.

Oh, damn it, not my soul for a hot fudge sundae. Please, no.

Baba, take this from me, please.

It goes away. It comes back. It comes back. It comes back. I arise, nod good-bye — I do not even do obeisance to the presence of Sai Baba in that living room.

I am on the streets again. To the nearest drive-in. So what if I'm alone? I eat them both, the banana split, the hot fudge sundae. I have them both.

Why do others get holy ash and I get empty ice cream dishes, and my lights on blinding, telling the waitress to come and clean it all up for me, I have to be on my way.

In the narrow room of self no prayer can thrive.
He who prays in suffering because of the melancholy which masters him and thinks that he prays in fear of God, or he who prays in joy because of the brightness of his mood and thinks he prays in love of God — his prayer is nothing at all.

For this fear is only melancholy and this love
is only empty joy.
— Martin Buber, quoting Zaddik in legend of
Baal Shem

(12)

"Marilyn, I can't go to conferences and seminars this
summer. I can't meet ten thousand new people."
"Yes, you can. Go."
"If I lose the weight, say 15 pounds, I'll go."
"Go no matter what. I think your passivity is most
of your trouble. You've stopped living. Your weight's not
changing and your mind isn't doing much either. Meditate,
pray, go to Huston Smith at Mann ranch and Jack
Schwarz in Oregon. Hell, it's summer vacation, isn't it?"
"Thank you, Sister."

(13)

I guess I'm ready. I fly to Oregon tomorrow. To five
days with Jack on "Transforming The Energies." I have
loaded my huge purse with candy bars — God knows,
they may not sell candy in Oregon.

(14)

Arrived today for Jack Schwarz's "Transforming the
Energies" Annual Conference. Mt. Hood, Oregon. The
green of Mt. Hood is itself a giant blessing. I have been
feeling better and better since I got here.
I arrived frightened that this time I might not find my
reaction to Yogi Schwarz favorable. So few things ever
are for me the same thing they have been before. But
I'm here now and the motel room has the same instant

adaptability to whoever I am as all the motel rooms of all my trips.

Now that I think of it, when I travel I'm like a motel room. As I get off an airplane I feel in myself the option of a new personality — as many new personalities as I might want. Things I would never say and do at home I do, say, and feel when I travel. It's not that the option isn't there at home, I guess — Jack would say there are nothing but options everywhere and you just need to find the one already chosen for you. I never do know who I'll be when I get off an airplane but this time I chose Miss Already Achieved Spirituality Girl. And I will not overeat!

Tonight was our first meeting as an assembled group. The one hundred and fifty or so of us met in the clubhouse (this is, of all things, a golf resort) banquet hall. We were seated at circular tables of eight. You got to choose, with registration, whether you were vegetarian or normal. I chose normal. I will eat what the people at my table eat and that will be that. It is again, as at the seminar, a varied group — students, teachers on vacation, doctors, church people, housewives. Everybody wants some of this consciousness.

There will be small group workshops going on for the largest part of the next few days, but tonight he spoke to us all, reassuring me immediately that I had been wise to come. He talked about what makes it possible to withstand what is for others pain. He had early in life discovered that he could ease pain by putting his hands over a person's body. He did not go about causing spectacular cures, but it was clear to him that he had a relationship with pain that others found difficult to establish. "Pain is an alarm clock. It awakens you to disharmony in body, heart, mind or soul. It says, 'Wake up, wake up.' But you don't need to hear the alarm clock ringing."

My 190 pounds — an alarm clock.

The evening brought us all together. I found it easy to talk to people. I walked back with Terry, who is in her thirties, what I call the "model" type, lovely face, thin body, stylishly dressed, gentle in her manner. She told me that she and her husband went to a healer in the Philippines because her husband had a tumor which was thought to be malignant. The healer, she said, heals by opening people's bodies without surgical instruments. He uses his fingers and pulls the skin open. Obviously this healer is a controversial figure. But Terry seems so sane and intelligent, it is hard to think she's reporting inaccurately. Her husband is well.

Terry left me at the cottage in which she is staying. I continued on in a soft drizzle. The evening had been exciting. As I neared my motel room I felt at one with the drizzle, the night smells, the world about me. Sometimes it is good to be rained on — tonight is one of those times.

Every minute that I am alone is like an extension of being with Jack and my thought processes seem to go on as he caused them to go on during the lecture. What did he say that cast the spell? I never remember. Tonight he talked in and about energy. "Instead of, how do I preserve human energies, ask a different question: how do I lose energy?" For Jack "patients" are people who have lost their energy or can't maintain it. Depression imprisons the energy. You haven't lost it; it's stuck in the unconscious.

I am a born "patient." I have been one so often.

It rained harder as I walked through the dark grass and up the stairs to my room. I went in and, before even putting on the light, came out onto the balcony. Black, deep night.

Some dark nights carry their own illumination. This seems to be one of them.

I suddenly see why I have been in so many difficulties whenever I tried analysis or psychotherapy. With a therapist I am a patient whose problems are all in her personal unconscious. So we attack the problem of my personal psyche. The analyst tells me to let go of the problems, free the personal unconscious. But I hang on.

With Jack, here, it is all let go. I feel so happy. All my fantasies are healthy. I am eating what everybody else eats. My problems drop away. I do not feel jealous or ferocious; nobody has to wait upon my moods. I relate honestly to people. Jack talks of a vortex in Oregon where the physical energy field around the area makes it a place of good energies. He is the vortex for me. I see that my cure will have to be a whole one.

The therapy message has been that my passivity has been based on a refusal to meet my problems. Tonight, when I heard Jack say, "Remember you are not just part of the universe, you are the total universe. Even if you are not conscious of it. Do not put limitation on yourself when you are both part and the total," I realized that my problems are not on the personal level. It never makes sense that I'm eating for this reason or that reason — there's never enough evidence to convince me of any theory any way. But tonight I feel that the demand is for me to change my life — not my way of thinking, not my unconscious conflicts, etc., but my very life — where I live, what I do, with whom, and in service to which god. So I remain passive, safe, and fat.

I stand on the balcony and think. I think, and all the fears come back. I want to eat. There is no place to go for food.

(15)

Woke to the mountains and trees and the rain they claim is inevitable and interminable. I love it. I glimpsed a cure for me this morning, in a dancing tree suddenly made into light. And then I went into the tree.

Had my first Tai Chi exercise. A leaning into, a leaning from, a blending of body and air. Lightweight, I moved in mist and morning. What a fabulous thing to do.

I stepped on my tall and handsome partner, but he buoyed me up, never changing his breathing, not wincing at this body bombarding him.

But breakfast came and went, grapefruit juice, one piece of bread, and jam and eggs and sausage: 650 calories — a day's supply. Oh, no, ho, ho, it's still me down here. Who can stay so high? Food Tai Chi is what I need to learn. Still, it isn't a binge.

> As long as you are capable of being offended
> you will need methods of defense.
> — Jack Schwarz

Today we talked about auras. Jack reminded us succinctly that to see another's field of energy you have to look out through your own. The window had better be clear. For a therapist to have the capacity to see your flow of energy, he must have his own energies right. If the therapist can see what's causing the blockage, you can peep over, or peek around. A doctor in the audience, an actual real life M.D. doctor, said, "Blockage is believing that 'more is better,' which is an American disease."

(16)

> You couldn't be closer to God than you already
> are. You're closer to God than your tongue to
> your palate.
> — Book of Mirdad

(17)

Eye Exercise

"To get at the pilot light of self, roll your eyes all the way up, looking back to top of brain. Then bring eyelids down but keep eyes upward. What do you see?"

I'm the kid who took college physiology, worked months with a microscope, got an A, and never once saw anything under the microscope. I can never do exercises of the simplest nature. Other people go right into alpha — not me, I'm in there thinking all the time. Hypnosis, light trance at best. But today I did it and saw a purple light unlike any I'd ever seen and a cylinder shape. I doubt that the eye exercise is calorically consuming, but it was nice to be able to do something and have it come out physically right. I have no idea what use the cylinder shape or the purple is, but I saw.

(18)

The most average middle-aged lady, well-groomed and well-mannered, whom I would probably never meet in any other way than this unusual one, this Mrs. W. levitates. She tells her story simply and unassumingly. It's just that once, during this prayer group meeting she and some friends have, she levitated. All in the group saw it. She was about six inches off the ground. Did she? I think she may have.

Oh, come on, Karen, nobody levitates. Yeah, I know, but I think she may have.

(19)

I was in Small Group Meditation with Terry this morning. Only six of us, in a circle, on the plush rug of the Winners' Trophy Room. We sat silently, listening to a tape that told us to go into the place in our head and find images there. Terry and I agreed beforehand to try to send each other's images to each other. We compared notes afterwards. We had both thought of the Taj Mahal and the leaning tower of Pisa. Doing that, and coming up with those images . . . what's next? I can't picture myself a psychic. Maybe I can just receive, from Terry. All the people here say they are undergoing transformations. To me they all seem to have arrived transformed. They look like me, but they all live in a different place from the typical American me.

I have such a long way to go to see people as people instead of all as pieces of a Freudian machine. My mind is a Freudian trap. When I feel God a voice says, "Substitution for security figures of childhood held by infantile inability to cope with reality principle." Garbage. I bought Freud thoroughly at 14 because I read a book that said if people tried to trick Freud, as they did at the beginning of his work on dreams, and told him a phony dream, he could analyze it as if it were real. That is, the made-up dream would have to be as relevant as the real dream. That took care of the creative act of the imagination for me. I bought it completely, breathed it in. I am a product of malfunctioning sexual libido. Damn, what a waste of years.

(20)

The quest is what makes the transformation. The transformation is what makes the quest. They are the same.

— Jack

(21)

Late night clear thinking: She must be the artichoke of the mother.

(22)

I am not eating or thinking about eating between meals.
I have a new energy. I am reading Hesse on my balcony
from 5 a.m. to dawn and writing after that. I am high
when I go to bed and high when I get up. Siddhartha
rings new and clear at this height.

> Where does it come from? he asked himself. What
> is the reason for this feeling of happiness? Does
> it arise from my good long sleep which has done
> me so much good? Or from the word Om which
> I pronounced? Or because I have run away,
> because my flight is accomplished?
> The river laughed. Yes, that was how it was.
> Everything that was not suffered to the end, and,
> finally, concluded, recurred, — and the same sor-
> rows were undergone.

I am Siddhartha and thin.

(23)

Let go and let God.

— Jack

(24)

Three days are already gone ... Other things go on
here besides lectures and meditations, but I have been
so full of books to read and ideas to write down that
I have not tried any of them. Tonight I went up to the
Jacuzzi to see if my new soul could reveal its old body
and just get up there, undress, and get in the water with
everybody. The round, heavy pool, the nude bodies,
unclear, but shaping water in a thin flow. I see that here
in this pool I am no new soul. I am what I can't get
rid of. Up here, in this water, we're all potential lovers

and my body is the story, not where my head is. I may be wrong, but I came back. I will rise up again into the trees and out onto the golf course.

(25)

Next morning. Woke to thoughts of Baba and of prayer. A form of dawn meditation: Seize whatever consciousness you have and program thyself. I did, in the presence of Mt. Hood, wake to prayer so that I could break the cycle. I did the mantra *Om Mani Padme Hum* and after each *om mani* I prayed and programmed: "I will throw up if I eat pancakes, sausage, or bread, ice cream or potatoes." I visualized throwing up. Maybe it will work.

Weight loss must be seen in terms of energy flow. I've been dead, so eating for proof of being alive. There is a Chinese restaurant near me which has over its doorway a sign reading: To Eat Is to Believe.

(26)

Enter voices.

I: Complex A, I've given you a lot of energy. You've run the show even, but that hasn't made you happy. I see you as a hurt child. You're always grabbing. How can I help you?

Complex A: Play with me. Use your imagination to give me a *safe* life. One reason I eat so much is because I go out there to get love but I keep losing it.

I: Maybe no one can get love. Only give it.

A: No, you can get it. It's just that I can't get enough and I can't let go of it. I've got stories for you to tell, truthful ones, of pain and of a sometimes magic that decays when the sleight of hand becomes too noticeable.

I: Well, I can't tell all your stories yet. I don't know that much. Isn't there something else I could do temporarily?

A: Meditate. I dig that.

(27)

Voices: Overeater, do not be misled. You are being asked to make a change at the deepest level of your being. What that change is must be a personal quest . . .

(28)

Got nauseated at orange juice. Drank it anyway. Nearly threw up. It works. The programming works.

(29)

.

Where did my eating like everybody else go? I'm eating everything in the communal dishes we have. I take the food first and then am reaching for a second helping just barely after the others get their first, and I do it all casually.

I am eating compulsively and thinking of suicide. I'm happy here. It's the kind of place I want to live in — not just the physical but to live with religious people, people on my trip. I've been having what I want this week and with loving people. If I can't make it here . . .

Later: Tonight, despite the eating, something happened to me that has never happened before. I walked into the dining room late and walked about looking for an empty seat, or for one of my friends. And suddenly I had a sensation I'd never had before. It was overwhelming and unfamiliar, and it was several seconds before I could distinguish that it was a positive feeling. Suddenly I knew. I felt completely at ease in this room with all these people. I have never had such a feeling before. I simply did not know what it meant to feel at ease in a group. With all my fat I stood there and felt loved and loving. I found a seat and ate a normal dinner. I huddled the feeling inside of me. When I got up to leave and walked from the dining room into the lecture hall I was again immersed in the new. A voice inside me screamed, "And you were going to kill yourself! To kill yourself when you're here and on this trip, when it's all about what you'll do with what you have. And you were going to kill yourself. That is sin."

When the voice stopped I knew that no matter what I eat, or weigh, or suffer for it, I will not kill myself over being fat.

Maybe.

(30)

Last day of conference. Damn, I must get to the real stuff. I sneak into the coffee shop, pray no one of the group sees me, order hot fudge sundae. Good God, what will I say if one of them sees me? Damn, this is a crazy sickness.

(31)

When you have been asking the same questions for years and not progressing toward any conclusions, you should decide one of two things. Either there are no answers to your questions or you have been going about finding the answers in the wrong way and something should be done about that.

(32)

Flew back to L.A. Feel like I'm in limbo, waiting to leave by car tomorrow to go up to northern California to Mann Ranch.

(33)

Buddhist Time with Huston Smith

The first time I ever heard of any Buddhist theory or belief, I was about fifteen and on the stoop of my house in Brooklyn. Somebody said, "'In Buddhism, they don't believe the world ever had a start or will ever end. They believe it always was.''

That was one of my bodhi tree enlightenments. Something that made sense. For I had spent enough time surely trying to figure out how the world could have had a beginning, but then how did God get there and how did He start, and where will it all end, and all of that questioning. I was ready to sign up for Buddhism.

Today that theory doesn't really seem as all-encompassing an answer as it did. It sure was a great clarification though. And a sense of attachment (forbidden) to it all remains.

It is easy to get into the sense of the spiritual here at Mann Ranch. The seminars are held in the living room of this magnificent old house, and the seminars and the ranch seem to have been made for each other. It is the only house for miles about, and though it is not a massive structure, it feels like a mansion. The living room is bookish, has old comfortable couches and a piano. Near the doorway is a beautiful brass gong brought from Tibet, years and years ago. It announces dinner times.

There are seminars on music, astrology, religions, everything, and I think there must be a layer of vibrations left from every seminar and these soak into the present weekend. All of the people, about 20 of us, are under the influence of this calm and radiant sense of place.

Also under the influence of the calm and radiance of Huston Smith. I'm in love with him already. He is a mixture of professor and impish boy. He and I each have a private room in the large house here, but on either side of a large bathroom which we are both to use. So we won't use it at the same time, each door into the bathroom can be locked from the inside. Huston keeps locking me out. He forgets to unlock the bathroom after he has gone out. I have taken to pounding on his door. We both think it's very funny and are planning a complicated series of knocks to use for all occasions. He is marvelously funny and marvelously brilliant. He wears his prominence as a world-scholar gracefully. He is very handsome but so warm that one is not put off by a fear of speaking to him.

We meet for sessions morning, afternoon, evening. He tells us about Buddhism and discussions go outward from there. Again I feel at ease in a group of people. The encounters here do not go for blood, they go for spirit, and I see what is missing from group therapies I have seen.

I was able to talk in the group about the tree falling in the forest and Krishnamurti's reason for the importance of not "retaining" what you learn. I was able to say that since I was 14 and first heard Krishnamurti I had hauled out from the back of my head to the front part at least two or three times a year all the questions he raised. I was able to say that I understand the importance of nothing except metaphysical questions. And I understand that those questions have no relevance to the people I know.

A woman, younger than I, said that ever since she'd been a kid she'd been concerned with a certain sense of the fear of death that was something different from what others meant by this fear. I sat forward on my chair. She said it was a certain falling into an abyss that comes on one. I would never have had the ability to say what she had said — I am always afraid to reveal the deepest scared parts of me. But I went to her and said, 'I know the abyss,' and there was nothing more that needed to be said. I don't remember her name or her husband's, but it was one of the most fortunate encounters I have ever had. Such encounters, one after the other, cannot be between fat and thin people, gay and straight people, vegetarian and nonvegetarian people. Those encounters bridge all the gaps and, in me, heal the gap.

Karen: This death thing comes and swoops — I am overtaken.

Therapist: That is your unconscious overwhelming your weak ego. Perhaps we can do something about that.

Karen: You mean you'll fix it so I don't have to die?

Therapist: Oh no, not that. We'll just give you a stronger ego.

Karen: It hardly seems worth the trouble, does it?

(34)

It is the kindest respite. I am eating far too much but only at meals. I am not racing about for hot fudge sundaes. (It's fifty miles of mountain curves from here to the nearest Baskin-Robbins, but normally I don't think that would stop me.)

I am being damned by my body, my uncontrolled and semi-real body. The day before I arrived I ate and then slept on the table in the local library, hand as pillow, the desire for tears as well as sleep nearly overwhelming. I do not want to miss a second and I miss hours.

There are four levels of Nirvana experience:

Level One: The stream winner, one who makes it across the River, Siddhartha. It is having had the glimpse. Once one has the glimpse you come back to it in life after life.

Level Two: Once-returner — one more life to go to make it to permanent Nirvana.

Level Three: Going to make it in this life.
Level Four: Realized soul — lives now in state of Nirvana.

Part of me knows that everybody is a stream winner. Everyone surely has had a glimpse of the reality of other dimensions. For me, I wait for the Nirvana of not wanting to eat.

The words "ultimate purpose" can recall me from anywhere. Huston speaks them from under the tree on the lawn in front of this old and magnificent house and I am recalled from a figureless daydream. Was I free and thin and running? Or numb from lunch? Things are spacing themselves weirdly. Something must happen.

(35)

Most of the people here make me feel that they do not see the weight. I see it. I cannot swim naked here either. There is a heavy woman here who can and dives in freely. I know her soul is in one hell of a good place. Mine is in hell. The most obvious evidence of my spiritual plight is my weight. This needn't be true for anyone else. For me the problem spreads out here like the Zen koans we have been talking about. It is real and definable and can be stated logically but not solved intellectually. I have mucked about in it psychologically, and I think it can only be solved religiously. I've thought this a lot lately, but nothing changes.

How does a nice Jewish girl wake up one morning and find herself a Christian? A Buddhist yet? Believing in Mara and in the devil?

(36)

What I see through all this love and life about me is that I am consumed by and consuming devils and they will not be got rid of once and for all and all at once.

(37)

Huston says that when considering the epics in every cosmic cycle we are today but a shadow of our full humanity of other ages. But everywhere we still carry within ourselves the full human capacity.

Enlightenment is not an emotional goal.

(38)

The criminally insane get away with it. What do the suicidally insane get?

(39)

Conversation after Huston Smith
Friend to me: Have you considered that no matter how wonderful and continually expansive the universe is, it is still meaningless to an individual?
K: Yes. In defense, however, I conclude: If you want to waste this trip, go ahead.

(40)

I cannot describe this, even for myself for that sometime later I always expect, in which I, wise and problem-solved, look back upon myself, bringing forth the great wisdom sucked from the pain. I ate all the way home. A twelve-hour drive became sixteen because I stopped place after place. I cannot record what I ate, where I stopped, how much I lugged into the trash can of my car — the car the first stop, my stomach the second. All light fell away. Philosophy cannot exist along with this monster that I am.

I cannot go on. I give up. Okay. I have heard that when you hit bottom you got to OA. I'll go.

(41)

Despair is the necessary prerequisite for each next step.

Part Three

Report from OA

When a wild elephant is to be tamed and trained, the best way to begin is by yoking it to one that has already reached that condition.

> — Huston Smith, discussing "Right Association" on Buddha's path.

Although we get few or no comforts here, we shall be making a great mistake if we worry over our health, especially as it will not be improved by our anxiety about it — that I well know. I know, too, that our progress has nothing to do with the body, which is the thing that matters least. What the journey which I am referring to demands is great humility, and it is the lack of this, I think, if you see what I mean, which prevents us from making progress.

> — Saint Theresa of Avila, *Interior Castle*

(1)

Mid-July

The church stands like a beacon. It is on the center of a major intersection, surrounded on all sides by thoroughfares. Episcopal Church of Our Saviour. Crescent Heights and Olympic. Overeaters Anonymous. They were listed in the phone book. I called and the girl who answered asked me where I lived and then told me to come to Crescent Heights at 7 p.m. for a Newcomers' Meeting.

The meeting itself is not in the sanctuary proper, but in an adjoining hall. It is a plain room. I enter and the first thing I see is a large sign that says: WE CARE. I walk in fast and take the farthest seat in the back row of the hall. Seated, I look around again. There are about thirty people, about twenty of us fat and the others in varying degrees of thinness (150 or so, I call slim). But I am not the heaviest person here. There are at least three people who must be in the 300s, and the other fat ones are somewhat heavier than I. I'm not out of place.

There is a table in the front of the room. It is bare except for an open looseleaf notebook on it, and within a few minutes of my arrival, this table becomes the focal point of interest. A thin, red-headed lady walks up to the front of the room, gets behind the table, places her hands palm down on the table, leans her weight forward and smiles out at us all.

"Hi, my name is Amy, and I am a compulsive overeater and your leader for tonight. Will you all join me in saying *The Serenity Prayer:* God, grant me the serenity to accept the things I cannot change, the courage to change the things I can, and wisdom to know the difference."

They all recited and I was able to join right in since the words were on the wall above the table. After the prayer, Amy went on.

"Several of us will share with you today and then answer questions you have. At eight o'clock there is a regular meeting and we hope you'll stay for it. You'll hear a lot of things in the meetings tonight. But I want to tell you the most important thing you will ever hear in OA. It is: *Keep coming back!*

"There are over two hundred meetings a week in the greater Los Angeles area and they are each a little different. But the basic program will always be the same. We follow the Twelve Steps and Twelve Traditions of Alcoholics Anonymous and in every way our program is the same as the AA program, except that we substitute the word 'food' for the word 'alcohol' when that appears in the Big Book of AA, which is called, simply enough, *Alcoholics Anonymous*. At the break you can look at it on the literature table in the back. We also use the AA book *Twelve Steps and Twelve Traditions*. Besides that, we have some special material printed by OA, and that is available to you for cost, as are all the materials on the table.

"As I say, there are two hundred meetings, somewhat the same, but also different. Some are participation meetings, where everyone shares his 'experience, strength, and hope,' and some are speaker meetings. Some are large, some are small. Some are in churches, some in banks, some in people's houses, and some, even, in restaurants."

(Everybody laughed and I felt a little more at ease. The girl had something about her of the recent religious convert. She had it all down pat and was eager to share it.)

"All of our meetings, large or small, though, begin the same way. I've asked Mona to read 'How It Works'."

It's hard for me to listen when people read at me, but I tried. My mind wandered, out among the fields and streams of sugar land, but came back and caught snatches here and there.

"Rarely have we seen a person fail who has thoroughly followed our path. Those who do not recover are people who cannot or will not completely give themselves to this simple program, usually men and women who are constitutionally incapable of being honest with themselves. . ."

"Half-measures availed us nothing. We stood at the turning point. We asked His protection and care with complete abandon."

"Here are the steps we took:

"1. We admitted we were powerless over food — that our lives had become unmanageable.

"2. Came to believe that a Power greater than ourselves could restore us to sanity.

"3. Made a decision to turn our will and our lives over to the care of God as we understood Him.

"4. Made a searching and fearless moral inventory of ourselves.

"5. Admitted to God, to ourselves, and to another human being the exact nature of our wrongs.

"6. Were entirely ready to have God remove all these defects of character.

"7. Humbly asked Him to remove our shortcomings.

"8. Made a list of all persons we had harmed and became willing to make amends to them all.

"9. Made direct amends to such people wherever possible, except when to do so would injure them or others.

"10. Continued to take personal inventory and, when we were wrong, promptly admitted it.

"11. Sought through prayer and meditation to improve our conscious contact with God as we understood Him, praying only for knowledge of His will for us and the power to carry that out.

"12. Having had a spiritual awakening as the result of these steps, we tried to carry this message to compulsive overeaters and practice these principles in all our affairs."

"I've asked Mark to share with us the tools of the OA program."

"Hi, my name is Mark." (He was about nineteen, round of face, fat of belly, sloppy, at least 50 pounds overweight.) "I'm a compulsive overeater. The tools of the program include: Abstinence, Sponsorship, Anonymity, Meetings, Phone Calls, Literature, and Service. We're going to explain these briefly and will answer questions you may have at the break."

The woman next to me leaned over and said, "I'm hungry, aren't you? When do they weight us?"

I smiled at her and quickly turned my attention back to Mark.

"Before I go on, I'd like to 'qualify.' I came into this program eight months ago, a hundred and thirty pounds overweight. I am now only fifty pounds from my goal weight and my entire life has been changed in this room.

"The first tool is Abstinence. This means a planned food program. OA is not a diet club and no specific food plan is required. There is no weighing in at OA. We are here to teach you how to abstain from compulsive overeating one day at a time, for the rest of your life. Our illness is physical, emotional, and spiritual. Losing the weight is only the physical part. Many of us have found that in order to maintain our abstinence we need to abstain from eating any sugars and starches at all, particularly all manmade refined carbohydrates. Some of us weigh and measure our food. Some of us do not have to do that.

"We suggest that you get a food sponsor and call in the details of your plan for at least twenty-one days. Will the qualified food sponsors in the room please stand?"

(I looked around. There were about fifteen women standing. All fairly thin, though only a few had probably completed their weight-loss program.)

"Besides a food sponsor, we have a step sponsor. Your step, or spiritual, sponsor will help you work the Twelve Steps of the program. It is the steps that help us stay thin."

Mark sat down.

Next a very thin girl stood up and walked to the front of the room.

"Hi, my name is Emily and I'm a compulsive overeater. Another tool of our program is Anonymity. This means several things. One is that what is said in the meeting stays in the meeting. This is not a gossip society, even though we hear an awful lot that's juicy enough to be worth repeating. People who come here need to be able to speak freely. Anonymity means also that if we meet a member on the street we don't introduce him to our friends as an OA member. It also means that we maintain anonymity at the level of books, films, or television or any other national level of publicity.

"Oh, I forgot to qualify. I came into OA three years ago at two-hundred pounds and have been maintaining an eighty-pound weight loss for over two years now. The program works."

"Hi, my name is Arthur and I'm a compulsive overeater." (Arthur is about sixty-five years old, gray beard and gray hair. Sparkling though.) "Meetings are a primary tool of the OA program. It is advised that for your first thirty days you go to at least five meetings a week. Some people find — to be honest, I found that I needed ten meetings a week. Now I only need four a week. That may sound like a lot of time loss but I was putting in at least that much time eating. I weighed three-hundred pounds when I walked in that door and that took a lot of eating time. Now I eat three weighed and measured meals a day, and I have maintained a hundred pound weight loss for two years. Plus I have more dates with lovely women."

(Weighed and measured fool . . . he's too old for me.)

"Hi, my name is Betty, and I'm an alcoholic and a compulsive overeater, and I'm going to explain the tools of Phone Calls, Literature, and Service.

"Phone calls are our meetings between meetings. We phone instead of taking the first compulsive bite which sends us off onto a binge.

"We phone our sponsors whenever we sense our compulsion coming on. And we phone to help others. And we stay on the phone until the compulsion to eat has passed.

"Literature — do yourself a favor and read the Big Book.

"Service — is what I'm doing coming here and speaking at a Newcomers' Meeting and sharing with you that I have lost sixty pounds and have kept it off for over a year. Service helps you hang onto your abstinence. Thank you."

She sat down to applause, as had the others. I'm getting the hang of it, you applaud whenever anyone speaks. Seems silly but maybe they know what they're doing.

Amy, the leader, went on. "Now I'd like to share with you my own story." She again identified herself. "We call it a pitch when someone stands up here to talk to us. Generally a pitch is three minutes maximum, but the leader gets a longer time."

The lady next to me got up and left.

Amy shared. Her background was very different from mine — she'd always been fat. She was in her late thirties now. Nobody really ever accepted her before OA, she said. A lot of what she said was about being fat as a child and that horror, and I didn't identify, but when she spoke of the bingeing that came just before she found OA, I knew I was home at last. She said, among other things, that in order to go to a job interview she'd take a half-gallon of ice cream with her and eat it, and drink the melted part, in a ladies' room before going into the office where sane people waited to judge her ability to do a job. She was an alcoholic eater, she insisted.

There was a lot of being saved by God in her pitch but also a pride in her voice which indicated she felt pretty proud of herself also. She concluded by saying that she has accepted that she cannot eat any sugar, barely one fruit a day even, and that she has to weigh out her four ounces of protein at every meal and will have to do so forever. "But," she concluded, "if I do these things, and work the Twelve Steps of the program one day at a time, I do not have to eat compulsively ever again."

Applause.

She said, "This is our break time and someone will talk to you if you have questions. After the break you will get to hear the regular meeting which begins in fifteen minutes."

I considered leaving. By this time I wanted my ice cream. Wonder where my fat lady of the next seat had gone first? Would I bump into her if I left?

I pushed through the bodies to get to the literature table. I bought everything.

Mark came up to me. "Hi," he said. "What's your name?"

"Karen."

"Are you enjoying the meeting?"

"Well, I don't know if that's the word for what I feel."

"No, I know what you mean. When I came here the

first time — hell, the first ten times, — I was scared to death of everything and everybody."

"I'm scared," I said.

He smiled. "Do you have any questions?"

I couldn't think of one.

He said, "May I have your phone number? I'd like to call you next week and see how you're doing. You might have some questions by then."

I gave him my number. "It's the first time anyone as young as you ever asked for my number."

"With our disease, all ages are the same."

During the break at least another thirty or so people have come in.

I sit down, putting my literature under the seat and sipping from a diet cola I'd bought from the All Diet soda machine in the back of the room.

The pitching begins. They talk, the volunteers or those who are called on, some casually, some emotionally, some enthusiastically, some as if they'd rather not be there. Very little is said about food. But I keep hearing about the weight losses and how long they've kept if off. I keep hearing about God, *The Serenity Prayer,* and spiritual revelations.

I couldn't sit through the whole meeting. The compulsion was too great. I left, out to repeat the actions which had brought me there in the first place. But as I made my first stop, Mrs. Good's for variety, I remembered what an AA friend of Marilyn's had told her about me and the possibility of OA. He had said, "She may not have hit bottom yet. When she has no other place to go, she'll go back to OA and it'll be all right for her."

(2)

Three days later

My phone rang.

"Hello."

"Hi, Karen?" (He sounded young.)

"Yes?"

"This is Mark from OA. How you doing?"

"Well, uh."

"Still out there doing it, huh?"

"Well, yes."

"Have you been to any other meetings?"

"No."

"Well, it took me a while to get started too."

"How long?"

"About fifteen years," he said. "Want some help?"

"Sure." (I had been eating raw meat when he called, waiting for the spaghetti and the sauce to be ready. And I knew what my night would be like. Devoted to the disease.)

"Okay. Will you do what I say?"

"Sure."

"Do you have any binge food in the house?"

They say the disease is "cunning, baffling, and powerful." Instinctively, I knew to lie. "Just some nuts," I said.

"That's not bad. Except you're probably lying. Why not throw them out and let me pick you up and take you to a meeting?"

"I can't tonight."

"Tomorrow night?"

"Busy."

"The next night?"

"You go to a lot of meetings, Mark."

"I want to keep my weight off. Besides, they're fun, once you get into them. Well..."

"Can I have your number? I'll call you, Mark."

He gave me his number. I wrote it down.

We hung up.

The sauce had almost bubbled over.

(3)

A week later

This morning I weighed 200. My sister-in-law said, "So, you've reached your goal weight. What now?"

I called OA again and found that again there was a night meeting at Crescent Heights. I was determined this time to give it a try. Otherwise it would be 210 the next week. I would get a food sponsor. During the day a sense of hope buoyed me up. Perhaps it will be the last triple cone. Perhaps not.

Tonight was far more religious in tone than I had even remembered, but it did not scare me away. Over and over again, in pitches, I heard, "You take what you want, leave the rest." I hung onto the pitches, listening carefully, waiting to find my food sponsor.

She found me.

I was standing alone during the break. I can usually handle conversations if others start them, but I am awkward at just going up to a stranger. She came up to me, fortunately.

"Hi, I'm Rhoda. Are you enjoying the meeting?"

"Yes," I said.

"Your first time?"

"Well, I went to the Newcomers' Meeting."

"Have you been abstaining since then?"

"No." (And then I blurted it out.) "I can't."

"That happens to a lot of people. You'll find it easier if you phone in your food."

Rhoda was elderly, sweet-looking, but at the same time something tough came across. She went on. "I used to drive to Santa Barbara just for a smorgasbord place there. Three ninety-five for dinner, a fortune in gas."

She looked like she wouldn't take any crap from a beginner.

"Rhoda, will you be my food sponsor?"

"Only if you're dead sure you're gonna do it. I don't like to waste my time."

I took her phone number, agreed to call at five to seven in the morning. (She has to stagger her calls.)

She suggested I paste the daily food plan onto my refrigerator door.

The meeting closed with the Lord's Prayer. It felt good. We all joined hands and said the prayer and after that "Amen" and "Keep coming back."

I came straight home. I did not binge. I will make it until morning. Will I call, I thought?

(4)

I did.

"Good morning, Karen. Right on time. What you going to eat today?"

"For breakfast, two eggs and an apple; for lunch, four ounces of cottage cheese, string beans, and a salad; for dinner, four ounces of lox, a bagel, a..."

She screamed, "What the hell do you mean, a bagel? Look, Karen, there are no bagels with me for a food sponsor. Do you understand?"

"Four ounces of hamburger, one cup cauliflower, two cups green salad with two tablespoons Roquefort."

"That's better. Karen don't come up with any more bagels. Why not a canary, for God's sake? Phone me tomorrow, or sooner if you have trouble. You don't have to abstain forever, just do it today. One day at a time. Go to a meeting tonight."

"Okay."

I pasted the words "ONE DAY AT A TIME" and the list of food I had called in on the refrigerator.

(5)

I made it through the day, through the meeting, through

the night. I have had a day of abstinence from compulsive overeating. I hesitate to feel hope. I've felt it at the beginning of days that ended buried under heaps of banana split. I hesitate to feel hope. My corny whipped-cream brain produces for me the image of a harbor. Yes. Harbor.

(6)

I have been to two meetings a day since my first day. I have four days of reported abstinence. Today at the meeting there was this huge circus fat man who went to the front of the church to pitch. He weighed at least 375 pounds. Everything about him was fat folding upon fat, but a beautiful face shone through what he described as the beginning of a spiritual experience — brought about by the abstinence which had already brought his weight down 75 pounds.

I think I've never before looked at a fat man's face.

(7)

Mentally, I'm feeling better, but physically —

> Like the other addicts, food addicts suffer from withdrawal symptoms. They have both physical and psychological reactions when their "normal" food supply is in any way curtailed. These can vary from imperceptible to very severe symptoms. They are sometimes mistaken for other illness. There may be digestive, respiratory, urinary, circulatory, and emotional disturbances in any number of combinations. There may be constipation, diarrhea, heartburn, indigestion, gas pains, spasms, cramps, air swallowing, urinary retention, urinary frequency, irregular heartbeat, rapid heartbeat, chest pain, shortness of breath, itching, etc., etc., as well as depression, anxiety,

irritability, fatigue, insomnia, excessive smoking, agitation, excessive worry, nightmares, unusual fears, etc., etc.

— Theodore Rubin, *Forever Thin*

With the exception of heavy smoking and insomnia, I have them all. Fun.

(7)

A twenty-eight-year-old girl, with, as they say, "a pretty face," stood up and told us of her life since nineteen — fat farms, diet pills, hypnotists. "Remember Mama Cass?" she said. "I always have that image with me." She started crying, running her fingers across her head, touching her long, beautiful hair — a gesture perhaps to comfort herself. Through the tears, we heard "I don't want to die alone, in bed, with a ham sandwich."

God, did I know what she meant!

(9)

I have eight days of abstinence. I am doing what they tell me. They talk about "working the Steps," that it is crucial to turn your will and your life over to the care of your Higher Power. For the atheists in the group — and there are quite a few — or at least quite a few who are vocal about this aspect of the program not being for them — for them the OA people say, "Pick any Higher Power you want. Some pick the ocean, some the group itself. One guy says Higher Power is the self he sees in the mirror."

They don't care what your HP is as long as you turn over your will, life, and food to that higher power. I haven't done that yet. I've picked the group as my HP and will do whatever it says until I get a step sponsor.

Maybe she can teach me the "turn over" part. That's obviously the secret here.

Then it's mainly you, the sponsor, and God.

In the meantime, I am joyous from not eating compulsively. If they told me to stand on my head four times a day facing east, I'd do it to the best of my ability.

For I am aware tonight, as I have been since that drive down from Mann Ranch, that much as I'd like to be thin again, it is much more a desire to be sane again. If I could only let the bagels go forever. Maybe I can. They say only a Higher Power can restore us to sanity. I'm listening, that much I can say.

It's an incredible feeling, not to be bingeing. It's a kind of relaxation period offered me after three years of jumping — failing to jump — the hurdles. Physically, I feel awful, but, if I can keep from that first taste of sugar, it will get better for me.

(10)

I have always had two distinctly different experiences of a blinding nature, ever since I was a child: an enormous sudden abysslike fear of death, and, at another time, an enormous sudden sense of the incredible miracle of life, of being here at all, of being able at such and such a point in time to be sitting eating two ounces of cheese. Tonight I had the miracle sensation again — to be sitting, fat, among peers, in an Overeaters Anonymous meeting, in a church in L.A.

(11)

Two weeks: My first crisis. People coming for dinner. An extra person coming I hadn't expected. I'll buy more Kentucky Colonel in time? I'll binge? That's it. There is no way to handle this situation other than to binge. The monumental problem of not enough chicken can be solved only by my bingeing.

I race to phone. I explain to Rhoda.

"When are they coming?"

"In an hour."

"Are you hungry?"

"Rhoda, at a time like this, could I be hungry?"

"Fine. Drink a diet soda. Do that now. Bring it to the phone."

"Okay, I've got it. I'm drinking it. . .I'm finished."

"Now, go get enough chicken for one more person. Take the compulsion with you if you have to, just don't order anything else. Write the order down on a piece of paper and give it to the man. Be a deaf mute. And call me when you get back."

Another day of abstinence. Is this the stuff that breaketh compulsion?

Heard: "Self-help is getting help from other people for your self."

(12)

Perhaps this is the place I can learn to be less shy. Of course, after you say, "Hello, my name is Karen, I'm a compulsive overeater," there isn't much left to be shy about. Everybody in the room knows immediately the worst secrets you have.

They say here that food is cunning, baffling, and powerful. It is helpful to me to put the reactions I have to food onto the food itself. It is enormously helpful to look at the food out there as some kind of magic essence, and once you reach to get the magic, you are hooked into reaching and reaching for more, and more, and with each bite the magical cunning moves about in you. It

will not be demagicked, this food. It will be respected.
It is cunning, baffling, and powerful.

Q. How can a Rocky Road ice cream cone be cunning?
A. Clever, isn't it?

Pandora's box was filled with fudge.

(13)

Annie, still remaining the nation's number one compulsively overeating dog, looks at me questioning as I
sit down to still another two pieces of chicken, broccoli,
and two cups of salad, barely grazed by two tablespoons
of Roquefort (sugar must be fifth ingredient on label of
bottle).

Her beige eyes query, "What has happened to the good
old days?"

With luck, Annie girl, the good old days are gone.

(14)

At last, a buddy. Alice and I went to a meeting together
tonight. That is we met outside the church and went in
and sat together. Alice, with bad teeth and not very pretty
to begin with, has more weight to lose than I do. We
came on the program almost the same day. Tonight we
were both close to going over the edge. Though we hadn't
said that. But you can tell, quite soon, not only about
yourself but about the other. And I care. I don't want
Alice to break her abstinence. I just don't want her to.
And I don't even know her last name, or where she works,
or how many children she has.

(15)

I am going to two meetings a day. That is about all I am doing. It's safest. I've been invited to coffee after the meetings but the group goes to Du Pars. Pies reflect too clearly in their glass cases. I am abstaining.

The smartest thing I have ever done was to give Rhoda my scale. I hear the weight losses daily — 10, 15, maybe 20 pounds a month is average at the start, then less. But I hear how long the people have kept their weight off since they lost it — 40 pounds, 50 pounds, 100 pounds — for six months, a year, five years.

I am advised to get a step sponsor, someone who will help me to work through the twelve steps. They indicate that working through the steps can take years — the rest of your life.

(16)

I have twenty-one days. This is the general period of calling in food, and for getting sugar out of the system. But Rhoda says she can tell I'm a tough case. Says I'd better continue calling.

I will.

(17)

Tonight it was there, full-blown. Right during the meeting — in the middle of the damn meeting. Eat, eat, get out of here, eat.

Then the voice of the meetings came in. "Just stay seated. If you're in a meeting you're safe." They tell you to bring the body and the mind will follow. Well, my mind is out the door miles ahead of my body. Oh shit, I don't want to start it all over again. Please.

Again I am invited to go to coffee, but I do not go. I may eat. After all, I have freedom of choice. My car, thank God, got me home. I called Rhoda. No answer — at coffee, doubtless, after some other meeting in some other part of the city. I called Ruth. I'd heard her pitch several times a week. She is tiny, looks like a swinger, a beach devotee perhaps, always healthy-looking. She weighed 325 pounds six years ago. They say to find someone who has what you want. I think she does.

I told her what had happened at the meeting.

"That's not unusual," she said. "Somebody must have said something about a situation which set off either your fears or your angers. Happens all the time."

"You're supposed to be safe in a meeting."

"A compulsive overeater is not now, not today, not tomorrow, not ever, safe; you'd better learn that fast. You are always to be an armed camp. It will come back. Set up phone call times, when you will call regardless of whether at that moment you are having trouble with your abstinence."

I am weary. It was a hard battle. "Do I have to do this every day of my life forever?"

"Yes, but only one day at a time."

"Thanks."

"Thank you for calling me. It works both ways."

Thank you, thank you, thank you.

I got into bed and the phone rang. It was Ruth.

"Are you praying?"

"No, I was having a hot fudge sundae."

"No, you weren't. I'd hear it in your voice. Do you pray?"

"I meditate."

"It's not the same thing."

"It'll have to do for now," I said.

Silence. "Okay. Finish your sundae."

(18)

"Came to believe that only a power greater than ourselves can restore us to sanity."

Who's not sane? I have just sat here for an hour, planning a Thanksgiving binge four months from now. They tell me over and over to turn the food over, get rid of it. They tell me everything. I nod my head, abstain today, and plan the binge. Why does it say "sanity" in that step? Isn't that a bit strong?

(19)

It's getting harder. They tell me it was a "honeymoon." Maybe I should not have stopped calling my food in to Rhoda. Alice is still calling in her food.

(20)

Extremely dangerous time. Visions of quarts of ice cream.

Let go, Karen; let go, Karen; let go, Karen.

I want to call up everybody I know and cry. I want my dead aunt Flo to come and visit me and cheer me up.

Abandonment — that is the feeling I am suffering. A speaker used the word tonight, touched the feeling, and I am enveloped in it. It is not a question of not liking friends but of fear of being abandoned by them. I would not be surprised if that is the root of the fear of death. Hang in, you weigh tomorrow.

(21)

Wow, 180!

(22)

My feelings are day-to-day crises. Hour-to-hour. Minute-to-minute. Tonight a man spoke to me. His name is Ed. We were at a participating meeting, where everybody gets to talk from a safe sitting-down position. I was off on the unfairness of God. Havoc wreaked upon the innocent. Why should one expect help with abstinence while cities shook and people starved? At the break he came up to me and said, "Hi, I'm Ed." (I knew who he was. He's blond and blue-eyed. Sydney was blond and blue-eyed. Somehow that gives a man an unfair advantage with me.) "Can I tell you two things?"

"Sure." (Just keep talking.)

"You don't have to run God's world, and you don't have to understand God's world."

I needed to say something to make him continue to be interested in me. Something fascinating. When I was thin I always said fascinating things.

"Oh."

He walked away.

Alice had heard his whole pitch at a speaker meeting. He has lost over 100 pounds and is also an alcoholic. He is married.

Down.

Tonight I felt exalted. Somebody said I was obviously doing well because I had stopped wearing one or the other of the two moo moo (that's how I spell it) sacks which appeared to be all I owned. Hell, I own more clothes than Elizabeth Taylor. That's all that could fit. I've a wardrobe in every size. Doesn't everybody? Didn't she?

It is less than twenty-four hours later and I am expected at Nor's for dinner. Maybe I should just stay at home and cook. She's a good enough friend to understand that I can't go out of the house because I might not arrive at the same weight at which I began my ten-minute journey.

This is where I'm supposed to call somebody. Who can I tell that I'm still so weak? Well, if I just don't eat, I don't have to call. It's funny but I don't want to give in a little — just eat a little extra.. It's the complusive all right. All or nothing. And no one has called me tonight. Abandonment.

"Hello, I'm Karen from OA."

"Hi, Karen, how you doin'?"

"Fine."

"Are you sure?"

"Oh yes, just calling to say hello. It says you should make phone calls. Right?"

"Right. Great. Hey, my baby's crying. You call again, okay? Right, 'bye. Keep coming back!"

Abandonment.

(23)

What is it that puts me far off about turning things over to God? Person after person at meetings pitches how God works their lives and programs for them. I have surely learned that What Have You exists; I have surely learned through meditation and study that I can tune into this What Have You. What is it that prevents good old positive thinking — the thoughts that will connect me directly to this Higher Power?

Perhaps that one doesn't want to get caught asking for something and then not getting it. And one knows better than to opt for a condition of man in which it is assumed everything is meaningful. Because if it is, why is everything such a fucking mess?

(24)

Dream. I am stabbed repeatedly with a large knife by a man who was trying to rape me. A psychologist? Then also another man — an intellectual that I wanted to take a course from — had attacked me. I fought for myself and think I was saved.

Dream. There were darling puppies, newborn, part beagle. I touched one. He flinched, was shocked. And then I realized he's never been *touched* before. As soon as he felt it, he loved it and was happy and cuddly and loving and wanted more. He'd become a real puppy.

The dreams stay with me. Once in a while one still needs to tip a hat to Freud. I woke from the dream remembering an actual incident, remembering the actual words.

It was shortly after my Aunt Flo's death. I was eating regularly, banana splits nightly, but I don't think I thought anything of it. Then, on this night which I suddenly recall but have never remembered before, I was coming home from somewhere with a girl friend. We were arguing about something (maybe even my weight gain, I don't remember) and she hurt my feelings. I got out of the car, in front of my house, mumbling a nonchalant goodnight, for it was not my way to show anyone they hurt me, and walking up those steps I thought, It's okay. All I have to do is keep eating and nobody can touch me.

And indeed they didn't.

Will I ever be a real puppy?

(25)

Of all places, at a small, usually comfortable OA meeting in a bank near my house, a mixed-up jerk called me a fat girl with dark glasses. I knew he was screwed up but he is skinny. So naturally I believed him.

I am not my body. Though I have known this since Jack Schwarz, I need to reassure myself daily that I am not my body. Nor is a man who is crippled his crippled legs. But we call him a "cripple." It is the tenet of the basic Americanism that that which is valuable is only that which is seen. I suppose that if we only judged others that way the greatest damage would not be done — we'd merely miss significant experiences, but if life is only a dress size anyway, what's lost? It is the pernicious judgment of ourselves that destroys us.

> It is no small pity, and should cause us no little shame, that, through our own fault, we do not understand ourselves, or know who we are. Would it not be a sign of great ignorance, my daughters, if a person were asked who he was, and could not say, and had no idea who his father or his mother was, or from what country he came? Though that is great stupidity, our own is incomparably greater if we make no attempt to discover what we are, and only know that we are living in these bodies and have a vague idea, because we have heard it and because our Faith tells us so, that we possess souls. As to what good qualities there may be in our souls, or who dwells within them, or how precious they are — those are things which we seldom consider and so we trouble little about carefully preserving the soul's beauty. All our interest is centered in the rough setting of the diamond, and in the outer wall of the castle — that is to say, in these bodies of ours.
>
> — Saint Theresa of Avila

Knowing that, have I got clear of it? How get clear? Seeing bodies remains seeing bodies. I remember the Brighton Beach locker room, where, at about the age of twelve, I first saw large groups of women of all ages naked. I remember looking and looking, and I had never seen bodies except girls my own age — not even my mother's — and I can still see in my head the lockers with clothes half in and half out, the people with clothes half on and half off and the cement covered by spread towels and that there were young bodies and old bodies, fat bodies and thin bodies. And the flesh of the old and the fat . . . hanging and ribbed, sagging, wrinkled. I remember thinking, How could anyone let her body get like that? My body could never be different from what it is today. And I remember turning away and never looking quite as hard, quite as broadly, quite as encompassingly, ever again.

(26)

Feel tonight that I've found a step sponsor, a spiritual sponsor. Ruth. I've talked to her before and tonight it sort of clicked in. Maybe she could tie together all the things that go pouring into my head from reading and from OA. She is in a place that mystics speak from, and I don't think she even realizes that. God came to her in a steady stream of light into a hotel room where she was experiencing fear. The light replaced the fear and has remained. She says to "affirm the Universe" — and means it. Not accept it, though she does. But walk around affirming it. She is living in the Light and feels we can all reach out to that and have it touch us. I believe her. Other than manifestations of metanoia, she does ordinary things like make a living in an ordinary business, buy flowers for the house, and books. I think the book thing made the identification for me. She quoted from a book that hadn't been on sale my first night.

> . . . You ran a race, you stumbled and fell, you have risen again and now you press on . . .: Do not stay to examine the spot where you fell.
> — *Twenty-four Hours a Day*

(27)

Alice has broken her abstinence. She pitched tonight. Says it happened four days ago. She said she doesn't

think she can ever get it back. Has eaten steadily for
four days, refusing to go out of the house. Her husband
has had to take the children to their relatives. He says
he will lock her in the bathroom if she doesn't stop. Her
face is already swollen, from food and crying. She stood
there crying, saying over and over again, "I want to stop,
I can't, I can't."

Then she ran out of the house.

"We'll never see her again," Rhoda said.

"How do you know?"

"I just know. After eight years I just know some
things. . . . Don't look at me like that, Karen. You'll make
it."

Okay, God, get out there on your charger and bring
Alice back.

(28)

I've already started having conversations with Ruth in
my head except I haven't had the courage to ask her
to make the commitment yet. She'd have to talk to me
every day. Look, ol' spiritual sponsor, ol' pal, you want
me to pray to a Higher Power. I just can't do that, not
on a personal, Help Me, level. What happens when I
put prayer on the personal level is not that my personal
experiences don't bear out a personal relationship with
God. A personal relationship with God. *Job* is clear
enough — that was his life, his relationship. His problem
was only to understand what his lack of understanding
had to mean in his life.

If I suffer, or even John F. Kennedy, God's Will can
be accepted — okay, I don't get it, but these things happening to me have a meaning, no doubt I deserve it,
or need to go through it or something, etc. What happens
to me, ol' spiritual sponsor gal, is that when I pray I

get visions of children starving to death by the 10,000's, concentration camps, and bomb victims. That's my hang-up, God, if you're listening. Every personal move I make of late makes God more than a force, it is clearer to me the Power I've believed in since my beginning to pay attention to altered states of consciousness. But the bleeding keeps getting in my way.

(29)

I'm hearing more of what is said at meetings. I'm listening better. There are two kinds of relationships that OA people seem to make to this Higher Power. There is a group, represented by the girl who says, "Since I've turned over my will and my life to the care of God, all my decisions are easy. I was in the market yesterday and couldn't decide which head of lettuce to buy. I listened for my inner voice and I know I picked the better one." (She's thin.)

And there is a group who have got ahold of something I think I'd like, a form of altered consciousness in which they seek not to get God to do their will, but to do God's will.

> "God, I offer myself to Thee — to build with me and to do with me as Thou wilt. Relieve me of the bondage of self, that I may better do Thy will. Take away my difficulties, that victory over them may bear witness to those I would help of Thy Power, Thy Love, and Thy Way of Life. May I do Thy Will always!"

Then they talk about the eleventh step. They also are thin.

(30)

Wednesday: Small group. A girl said, "I'm turning over parts of my life to the will of God, but I don't know how to turn the food over to God." I said, "Forget it. God doesn't eat refined carbohydrates."

Talked to a new member. I wanted her to come back. That's a great feeling. Feeling you have something to eat. Wow, "eat" was a great little old Freudian slip in there. Something to "give" that would truly be helpful.

I caught a guy looking at me in the way guys used to look — that was nice.

(31)

I have called Alice four times. First her husband said she wasn't home. The last time he said she told him to tell me she didn't want to speak to me or anyone from OA.

Vision. The Cosmos: See it push your sight out farther and farther.

Vision. Cheesecake.

Assignment. Compare. Do not intellectualize. Just look at them both. Compare.

(32)

The smallest pants in Lane Bryant were too big for me. Size 32 pants.

(33)

During a hard time I called Ruth. I told her I had to eat. There's no meeting for four more hours.

"Look, Karen," Ruth said, "choose a place on the floor. Sit there and try this. Let the compulsion rush or creep onto you as you sit there. Say a mantra or the Lord's Prayer, or the Shema, or breathe deeply. Stay there, damn it, keep your legs and feet and bottom and top, keep them there. Keep yourself there.

"*Remember this:* There is no place for a compulsion to go but away. If you can hold your ground long enough it will leave you. I'm not talking about a facile victory. It may be there for twenty hours at a time and you may wake up to it next morning, yet it will finally go, because it has no place to go to rest and sometimes you do have to have a place — God, or a friend."

I did it. First the food trucks rolled over me, then a feeling of terror. I started the Shema going in my head: "Hear, oh Israel, the Lord is our God."

Over and over. Then emptiness.

Falling and falling and no place to land.

Switched to the Lord's Prayer.

Noted that I should learn what a Hail Mary is. Approved of myself for making jokes while the armed battalions came out against me.

Suddenly, intense exhaustion. And a sense of calm. I have been in a wicked forest and I have come out. Serenity.

(34)

If it weren't for cantaloupe I don't know what we'd all do. It's the only food God has given woman that's as good as the bad stuff and not fattening. It'll probably turn out to cause cancer.

(35)

Last night with my ten-year-old niece I almost cheated. For the ultimate in sabotage you must set up people who do not know you're in OA, who think you just need to cut down, etc. She's a child, what does she know? Last night we were at the Golden Temple of Conscious Cookery. "Let Aunt Karen have a taste of your cheesecake, baby." I reached over. She jabbed her fork into my hand. "No," she said.

(36)

That little reach for the cheesecake terrifies me. I must be doing something wrong. Steps. Damn Steps. I need a step sponsor.

(37)

Panic sense. I'm old. There's no way for me to make up all I've lost.
Voice: That's true.

(38)

Dream. I am on a Ferris wheel. It goes out of control and I fall from my seat. By a miracle I am saved. I stay conscious and fall into the next empty seat.

(39)

I am not my body.

(40)

Hey, my underpants are loose.

(41)

Sponsor's Tale
"It can only have been you, Ruthie."

"No, I didn't."

"You're six years old and already you steal."

"No, I didn't."

"Ruthie, there's no one here but you and me. You stole the chocolate-covered Easter Bunny. Otherwise it would still be there next to the milk. What did you do with it?"

"It was chocolate all the way through," Ruthie said.

(42)

I've learned something from the pitches that simplifies hurting people. If you don't like someone it's very easy to hurt them: just tell them you don't like them and wish them great suffering and pain. That's all it takes. You don't even have to yell it. Just tell them, in a nice, calm voice, "I don't like you and I wish you great suffering and pain." That's all it takes.

And when I was a kid, I used to think up ways to get even with people!

(43)

Conversation with Ruth

"Karen, do you take the first three Steps every day?"

"I take One and Twelve."

"One and Twelve was your OA honeymoon. Without Three you can forget it. You wake up, you admit you're powerless, you realize that only a Higher Power can relieve you of your insanity, and you turn your will and your life over to that Power."

"How do you turn it over?"

"You'll learn, if you keep coming back."

"I know the slogan, Ruth. To be honest, I'm not sure God does such a good job with the cases he does get."

"Try it, try God."

"That's like a paid commercial on a TV show dedicated to violence."

"Try it, smart mouth."

(44)

In Ed's pitch

Do not listen to people who say that compulsive over-eating is only in your head. This can put you right back out there in the drive-ins. It can lead you to a "sophisticated" first bite. (If it's not physical, I can do it just for today. I've conquered it psychologically.)

"There are also lunatics who think alcoholics should learn to drink like normal people. I've at least not heard anyone say an addict should take heroin in small amounts to prove he's cured. People will assure you over and over again that sugar is a psychological addiction. Maybe. But those are not the rules of the game for the sugar-compulsive overeater.

"Try not to hate people who understand nothing about your disease. Just don't listen to them."

(45)

I heard today that Kevin, the circus fat man I had thought so beautiful, died in his sleep last night. He had months of abstinence and had lost over 100 pounds.

His heart just stopped.

(46)

Tonight I made a major step. Overheard Ruth say that she was speaking in San Bernardino tomorrow night and was having car trouble. I pushed into the conversation, "Could I drive you? I'd love to drive you." And she agreed to let me take her.

Well, I've been to San Bernardino and back. In the car going out the first thing Ruth said was, "Forgive me, but I get nervous before I give a forty-five minute pitch, so I'll probably not talk too much."

We drove almost in silence. I began to wonder if maybe on the road back I could ask her to be my step sponsor. I had considered asking Rhoda, but she had probably seen it coming and kept mentioning how many "babies" she had. What if Ruth had too many?

Her pitch was great. I taped it.

Hi, my name is Ruth. I'm a compulsive overeater. I came in at 325 and now weigh 125 and my weight sometimes fluctuates up and down 10 to 15 pounds. But I never break my abstinence from sugars and the rest takes care of itself. . .

This program promised me that I would come to know the words serenity and peace. It's difficult to explain why I didn't have it. I'd been running and while I was running I wasn't sane. I sought love and approval and I found it and it wasn't enough. In my seeking I sought acceptance and self-worth and I found it and it wasn't enough. So in the course of running I had to find something to fill the void I felt and my escape was food because I could shut off feelings of hurt and rejection and pain. It took what it took to get me here, all that food and all that weight and all that lack of self-approval to get me here. I came through the doors of OA a hopeless woman. I had nothing to live for. I didn't want to live and I really didn't care that much. I was told I would die and I didn't want the final humiliation of being buried in an oversize casket. Those were the feelings I felt that got me here.

What I found in OA is the simple word of hope. People who also looked all their lives for love, acceptance, happiness. I was not alone; all of us used food because it was the best we could do. OA said that if I came to you you would do for me what I was not able to do for myself, and together we would do it. It kept me coming back.

You presented me with tools and steps to recover on. I looked for peace and serenity and they were all just words, but the loving fellowship kept telling me to keep coming back — go on, things will get better. They did. Then I found what I had been looking for all the time — God. If I turned myself over to God I would get all of everything I wanted. I worked very hard at this because I wanted what everybody around me had. At last, through abstaining and using the tools, I began to feel it and to live it. Serenity is with me most of the time without my asking for it. I can walk down the street and no longer feel separate. I belong at last. I never have to be alone again. I thank God that it took what it took to get me here. It will all be there for you too.

I waited while everybody crowded around her after the meeting, and then it was over and we were outside.

"Glad that's over," she said, sighing a deep sigh, breathing in the fresh night air of San Bernardino.

"You didn't seem at all nervous."

"So they always tell me," she said and laughed.

We talked now on the way back. She told me about meeting Alan at an OA meeting shortly after she had lost her weight. They were married within two weeks and have been married four years already. It was a second marriage for them both.

She had led the meeting and Alan had been the speaker.

"Just substitute the word food whenever I say alcohol," was the usual opening line for an AA speaker.

I told her some more about my life, my marriage, my teaching — but we were practically back in L.A. and I still hadn't asked her. Come on, kid, come on.

"Ruth," I paused. (If she says no, it's because she has seven-hundred babies, don't feel bad.) "Would you be my step sponsor?"

"I thought I was," she said, laughing.

(47)

In all these eight weeks, in which I have lost 35 pounds, I had not pitched at Crescent Heights. There are always too many people there. And you have to speak on your feet in front of EVERYBODY. But tonight I raised my hand, got called on, and walked, trembling, to the front of the church hall. To my amazement a lot of people clapped as I went forward. I guess they'd all noticed I'd never pitched. It made me feel very much like an insider, a lady who "belonged."

Karen's First Pitch in Front of Everybody at Crescent Heights

"Hi, my name is Karen. I'm a compulsive overeater."

("Hi, Karen," they all greeted me.)

"I want to tell you what happened to me tonight before the meeting. Now that I've lost enough weight only to be fat, instead of gargantuan, I took the chance of going out into the real world. I went to a party at my friend's house." (They are all looking at me. . .they care.) "You know what I wore? Right, a black pants suit." (They are laughing. They know. They all have black pants suits, even the men.) "And this is the hottest August on record, right?" (This is less horrible an experience than I expected, this pitching.) "But I wouldn't take off my jacket, right?

The temperature in the room must have been 620 degrees. I was drenched. But I would not take off my jacket. No one in the room was going to see my arms. Not even if it killed me. On the desert with Lawrence of Arabia, I wouldn't take off my jacket. I wouldn't want a camel even to see my arms.

"Finally I got out and got here. Without having eaten anything on the goody table." (They clap. Giddiness overwhelms me. I say one last thing.) "Here, I can take off my jacket."

I do and go toward my seat, to great applause and laughter.

"Oh, what beautiful arms," Ed says, leaning backwards as I sat down.

I just happened to be sitting behind him.

(48)

I weighed today. Down to size 18 at Ohrbach's.

(49)

September: I abstain, I talk to Ruth, I talk to Newcomers' Meeting. I don't know how to "turn it over." Sometimes I think I have it for a second, and then it's gone.

. . .Every religion says that its method is the way and no other method will do. . . . Every method is just a device; it is just creating a situation for the happening. It is not causing it.

For example, beyond the boundary of this room is the unbound, open sky. You have never seen it. I can talk with you about the sky, about the freshness, about the sea, about all that is beyond this room, but you have not seen it. You do not know about it. You just laugh. You think

I am making it up. You say, "It's all fantastic. You are a dreamer." I cannot convince you to go outside because everything that I can talk about is meaningless to you.

Then I say, "The house is on fire." This is meaningful to you. This is something you can understand. Now I do not have to give you any explanations. I just run. You follow me. The house is not on fire, but the moment you are outside you don't have to ask me why I lied. The meaning is there. The sky is there. Now you thank me. Any lie will do. The lie was just a device; it was just a device to bring you outside. It did not cause the outside to be there.

— Bhagwan Shree Rajneesh

(50)

It is early September. I am getting up earlier every day, getting ready for work. School starts in a few weeks. How I hate for this period to end. It is so good not to have to concentrate on anything but my abstinence. They say, "Keep it simple," and so I am. Except for my interest in Ed. They say not to get involved romantically with anyone for the first year of abstinence. Who's getting involved? I'm lucky if I see him every other meeting or so.

I've never led such a repetitive, disciplined existence before. Breakfast, straighten up, meeting, lunch, read, go to park with Annie, make OA phone calls, dinner, go to meeting, occasionally have coffee afterward, come home, walk Annie, play Ping Pong kitty ball with Hepburn. Go to sleep. Every day.

Plus seizures of wanting to get out there and

eat up the city, and waiting out the compulsion, and phoning, instead of taking that first compulsive bite.

Sometimes the seizures are of anger. Today. I drove about the city, crossing and recrossing old binge routes, feeling surges of anger, hate, and resentment all at one time. It is not directed anywhere, except at me. It is just beating there in my head. I remember what Theodore Isaac Rubin said in *The Angry Book:* that it is a slush pile, all the resentment from babyhood on. He must be right because the anger has no visible content. It just goes on. Yelling and screaming and driving helped. I didn't eat.

(51)

School
"Oh, and how did you do it, Karen? You look wonderful."
"Overeaters Anonymous."
"Oh, really? Does it work?"
"Well, look."
"Well, Karen, anyone can take it off. Can you keep it off?"
"Good question. Try not to offer me any goodies."
"It's just a question of will power."

Terror.

(52)

I can see that it will be a year to tax our patriotism. For our Bicentennial celebration we are going to involve every child, teacher, and parent in a meaningful American experience. Culminating in a 200-candle birthday cake on a day-long program in the auditorium and in the yard.

Nine months to the birthday party and I'm worring over how to resist the cake. Would Uncle Sam be insulted if I abstained?

Children are the only thing that remain constant across the centuries, I'll bet. They may get different by the time they reach adolescence from century to century, from culture to culture, but there's still a joy in the package that is a first-grader which I'm sure has been there since the first school.

"Who's *your* teacher?"

(53)

Ruth: Keep a journal. Keep it by your bedside and write in it every night and morning. Write anything — what you did today, what you ate, who you resent, who you love. Start sentences with "I didn't want to eat that stuff an hour ago. What happened in the past hour?" Write down everything — what you were thinking about, to whom you spoke. Everything, and you may find out the reason for that particular compulsion at that particular time.

I've started it, but it doesn't seem to be too useful. I want to eat over every feeling. Pleasant, unpleasant, it doesn't matter. Once addicted, I think the whole system changes. An addict just wants his drug — good, bad, meaningless. The ego becomes totally one with the compulsion. The compulsion-addiction comes about in an act by ego to relieve itself from some pressure at the moment unbearable. It works and the behavior is started. The behavior is started and soon there is the addiction.

The only way to overrule the compulsion is by the numinous experience. Therefore the numinous must be strengthened all the time for it to play by itself, as an act of grace.

(54)

Complete inactivity due to Ed fantasies. I'm already into living together, running off. All he's done is be nice to me. But my mind can go, fueled by only one word of encouragement (say — "hello"), to "He'll leave his wife for me."

Today is my ninetieth day of abstinence. I pitched today at a Newcomers' Meeting. I told them how I ate until seventy days ago.

I told them how I ate one night, all sugar, all alone in my apartment, and suddenly it was morning. I'd slept with my head on the kitchen table; an unfinished doughnut, the last one, remained. Once you eat until you pass out, nobody can do other than equal you. You've reached the summit and the nadir at the same time, and you can do that over and over again. I got fatter, of course, but passing out is passing out and is sufficient for anyone as suicidal as I was.

Three people came up and thanked me for sharing. They too had eaten until they passed out.

> Sugar
> Is the trigger
> To make you bigger
> Fuck the trigger
> Fuck the trigger

Compulsive's Competition
> Put adjacent words to music,
> preferably something
> calorically consuming
> danceable
> enhanceable
> you.

From OA

I can put you up or I can put you down, but as long as I am comparing myself to you, I can't come out feeling good.

* * * *

When all else fails, try following directions.

* * * *

You happen to be a compulsive overeater. How many times before you know that any impulse to market at other than a previously planned time is a binge warning? No matter what you think you may need.

* * * *

If you speak the truth you're interesting. The truth you tell may be narrow and confined but it will be interesting.

* * * *

Resign from the debating society.

* * * *

The best way not to eat is don't.

* * * *

If it works, don't fix it.

* * * *

Bring the body and the mind will follow.

* * * *

Don't get involved romantically with anyone on the program in your first year.

(55)

Went with Helen and Dan to Port Hueneme, a favorite spot of theirs up the coast. Lovely ride up with Helen's brother, Aaron, except for an incredible memory that I had completely forgotten. It came upon me as we passed the Sears on 101 before Camarillo. Once, when Helen and Dan lived in Camarillo, in my bingeing years, I had eaten my supplies of everything and had not arrived. I had pulled off the highway, gone into Sears, bought $10.00 worth of candy on my credit card and taken it all into my car.

I began to eat the chocolates and the nut fudges and the marshmallow goodies. I think I wanted to get it all in my mouth before I reached Camarillo, fifteen miles farther.

The next thing I knew I was in the outskirts of Santa Barbara, thirty miles farther than I had to go. The alcoholics call it a blackout. I chose to forget it. But, passing Sears today, the terror of that awakening near Santa Barbara — I had not missed a turn or overshot my mark. There had been no highway, no mark, no turns. Just a lot of luck that I was still in my car, on the road, when I came to.

I shuddered. This time I got there right on time with Aaron.

Despite my recollection, or for whatever reason, when we set out for dinner I saw that I was in for hell. There was first the fact that I wanted to eat. I was hungry.

Also lots of fun food times in past with Helen. They suggested Chinese food. I actually said no — I couldn't think of resisting everything while perhaps munching a sparerib. They suggested McDonald's. I said please no. Okay. Then they suggested a shishkabob place. Only a prima donna could say no again. I felt trapped and slipping.

Menu came. No à la carte on menu. I just couldn't make a fuss and of course wanted all the trimmings, sourdough roll filled me with a depth of yearning I might not even be able to muster for Robert Redford or Omar Sharif. I made a head trip to Ruth and tried to explain to her that I had had no choices. She answered that it was the wanting and not the menu that was doing me in.

The waitress came. We asked if there was an à la carte menu. She said no, and I salivated. Then she said, did we want to see the sandwich menu? I saw my chance and knew that it was then or never.

I said I'd order from the sandwich menu and that I didn't think I needed to see it. Just a hamburger patty, please, some tomatoes, and a small green salad. They wanted dinners and ordered.

Triumph.

Then back to the motel — everybody's eating graham crackers. Damn, is it always going to be like this? Yes, Karen, no more fun with food ever. Look at all these normal people, eating what they want because they feel like it, and I, I'll never be normal about food. The "poor me" song played loud and clear. Then it struck me that Aaron, who could get graham crackers and ice cream, and etc., is blind, and that he was blind yesterday and will be blind tomorrow. And I doubt that he spends his day bemoaning his lack of normality. Dear Aaron, may you have graham crackers forever, and may I grow up a little some day or other.

There is a story from the time of Buddha of a beggarwoman who was one of the poorest beggars in India, because she was poor in kind and also poor in mind. She wanted so much and that made her feel even poorer. One day she heard that Buddha was invited to Anathapindika's palace in the Jeta Grove. Anathapindika was a wealthy householder and a great donor. So she decided to follow Buddha because she knew that he would give her food, whatever was left over. She attended the ceremony of offering food to the Sangha, to Buddha, and then she sat there waiting until Buddha saw her.

He turned around and asked her, "What do you want?" Of course he knew, but she had to actually admit and say it. And she said, "I want food. I want you to give me what is left over." And Buddha said, "In that case, you must first say 'No.'

"You have to refuse when I offer it to you." He held out the food to her, but she found it very difficult to say no. She realized that in all her life she had never said No. Whenever anyone had anything or offered her anything she had always said, "Yes, I want it." So she found it very difficult to say no, as she was not at all familiar with that word. After great difficulty she finally did say no and then Buddha gave her the food. And through this she realized that the real hunger inside her was the desire to own, grasp, possess and want....

— Chogyam Trungpa,
Cutting Through Spiritual Materialism

(56)

Am finally calling Ruth more regularly. Every time

I think I'm making it through, the beast stirs in me. But now I call before most of the suffering.

Ruth: Do you still have the feeling you need to eat compulsively?
K: Well, a little.
Ruth: I'm not getting off the phone until the desire to eat compulsively goes away.

Ruth said tonight, "How long do you want to feel bad? Set yourself a time and stick within it."

(57)

People's pains are specific. There is no such thing as a generalization, "pain." Remember that when you tell somebody you understand his suffering.

(58)

I've had life all wrong — permitted myself, out of an ass-backwards vanity, far too great a degree of suffering. The weight I carry may be a large and painful burden, but miracles are happening every day. It becomes irrelevant to be sick, to be in pain, to have an uncontrollable addiction to suffering. I hear a tyrant in me who says, "Kill yourself." But I don't have to kill myself. Other voices say, "Life," and I have to get into the space of those other voices.

(59)

Mike Douglas Show Fantasy

M.D.: Well, surely you're not a compulsive eater now.
K.R.: Yes.
M.D.: Look, you may have been a compulsive eater once,

but not now. I mean look at you — let's have the camera move in here on the slim lines of Ms. R's body.
K.R.: (smiling, trying to see self in camera): Would you tell a man who said, "I'm an alcoholic" that he isn't?
M.D.: Depends on could he walk straight.
K.R.: Sober twenty years. Alcoholic or not?
M.D.: No. Not.
K.R.: All you famous TV people are the same. No feeling for the common man.

(60)

Remarks to Hostesses
Hostess: You really didn't look to great, Karen. Being that heavy, you know.
K: How good of you never to mention it.

(61)

. . .Dreyfus assumed that acute traumatic experiences might influence the hypothalamic regulatory mechanisms, without bringing evidence in support of this. In my own observations, obesity develops not infrequently after the death of a family member, separation from home, when a love affair breaks up, or in other situations involving the fear of desertion and loneliness. Reactive obesity is the form more commonly observed in adults. The obesity seems to develop in response to an emotional trauma, frequently to the death of someone close to the patient or when the fear of death or injury is aroused. Overeating and obesity appear to serve the function of warding off anxiety or a depressive reaction.
— Hilde Bruch, *Eating Disorders*

Flo? Not Sydney? Hm-m-m. I must think about that. Again I see that place I so often get to when trying to figure out what went wrong with me somewhere, or what's wrong with some situation: there are too many variables. No matter how I try to exclude some and include others, in any human situation, I end up not being able to do the scientific method. It's Somebody's Sense of Humor, I guess.

(62)

Where does a lion sleep when he's in the house?
Anywhere he wants to.
How do you talk to God?
Politely.
God, have I got a long way to go?
Yes!
At last I've found God.
Now can I eat pumpkin pie?

(63)

— You got cured?
— For the time being, I seem to have. I'm thin.
— How?
— I told my secret.
— What was it?
— That doesn't matter.
— You mean you're not going to tell us the secret?
— No. Just imagine the one you have — that'll do for both of us.
— What is it? Come on.
— I'm serious. I learned something more important than how to tell my secret. Instead of my telling you my secret — for I no longer have need to tell you — you tell yours

to someone; yours is the more important secret now, not
having been told.
— But I have no secret.
— Bullshit.
— I don't.
— It's the nuances. Tell the nuances, the thinking that
went with the deeds. You've told the deed, maybe. Maybe
you've no secret deed, even, though I doubt that, but
you know what you need to tell. I know that you need
to tell it.
— If you want to know, I've been to a psychiatrist.
— Bully for you. Look, you have to tell your secret to
someone for free.

(64)

Why do I like gossip so much, always want the inside
story, want to know about the *real* lives? Because by nine
years old I knew that the secret life was more interesting,
stranger, and more unlikely ever to be known than the
life the world sees. Listening at OA confirms it. I am
a *voyeur*, that is all.

(65)

A lot of people talked about their mothers tonight.
I want to say something here for my mother. She taught
me that God is everywhere and in everything. She taught
me that I have never thanked her. Mother, I thank you
now.
Also, she said, "I always knew you would be bad."
"From when did you know that, mommy?"
"From when you were five."
Mommy, who isn't bad?

(66)

Tonight I see the root of it all. All I need to do is stand up in front of the OA group and say "I'm lonely" and I will be saved. Instead, I'm planning to binge.

One thing about compulsive eating — it sure makes you self-sufficient.

Blind is blind, unconscious is unconscious. Do not be misled. You will never know what is going on down there. Others will know about you — they see one person. You experience so many selves there is no hope to decipher yourself.

I buy two books and think, okay, so my emotional life is zero. But my intellectual and creative life goes on. And my spiritual life. As if my spiritual life was taken care of because I am not hurting anyone at this given point in my life. That is not the spiritual. The spiritual life is to be led by engaging in the spiritual tasks God sets for you. And God does set spiritual struggles before you. To ignore them is to neglect them. To neglect them is to proceed in the world at your own peril. I am realizing this and yet planning to conk out.

(67)

Why are there so many "roots of it all?"

Wanting to stay alive is a form of worship.

(68)

You're supposed to make phone calls when you are about to fuck it all. Work the program. If ever, now. Before you eat.

I dial Ruth. "What's up," she says, and I say, "Where is everybody? Where is everybody?" I keep saying it over and over again. I'm not even sure whom I mean, but Ruth seems to be all knowing.

She says, "There, they are there, they will be there."

I think I meant where are the people who will love me.

The binge feeling went away. So it can go by speaking the truth to someone.

That sounds easy, but most of the time I don't know what the truth even approximates. I have trouble telling the truth to a question like, How are you this morning? I consider what the answer should be. Maybe it is simpler, though, than I have thought. The truth is whatever you have just said to somebody that made the binge compulsion go away.

(69)

When I came home today from school the phone was ringing. I dashed in. It was Ed.

"Hi, just called to say hello. How's your abstinence?"

"Fine." (Oh, hello, hello.)

"What meeting are you going to tonight?"

"Crescent Heights."

"Maybe I'll see you there. 'Bye, Karen."

Maybe he'll see me there.

(70)

5:49 a.m. Thursday morning
Woke a few minutes ago singing in my head:
    something to dance about
    something to sing about
    to a fox trot or a waltz

I guess I know what it is about. In the beginning was Ed.

He talks program but it is walking with him that is doing me in. Levis. He thinks I look great. He admires me for working a good program.

(71)

I spent the night at Ed's, sleeping over. Being held all night, but not made love to. I told him the story of my life I guess that's an inventory all right. He told me to forgive myself. He told me his life story. He's in love with Judy. Which is nice, since she's his wife and is in Bermuda with the kids. And will be home any day now. She understands his work in OA and AA. Was an alcoholic but never fat.

Could God have given me anyone else more perfectly suited to heal me? That damned first analyst I went to could never have done it. He just wanted me the same as the rest of the men in my life. Some blessing. Ruth couldn't have done it because she's a woman. And Ed couldn't have done it if I hadn't known that he did want me physically. And loves me as he does all OA people. Not having me, he saved me. It was an incredible feeling, being held that way. Tears against our cheeks. And almost crying.

I think last night was the best sex I've ever had, and we didn't even screw.

Since I have come away, though I have had the urge to eat, as I can't turn it over to God, I am turning it temporarily over to Ed. (Till he meets Judy at the airport?) Maybe I want to eat out of happiness. It's there no matter where I turn, the monkey.

But it's becoming a somewhat different monkey.

He gave me so much, such a calm sense of love. I'll never be in love desperately again. Followed by, I'm desperately in love with Ed, but I'm not. I love him, but I'm really ready to accept my being an OA baby to him, and leave it at that. For now.

(72)

The compulsion is awful. Not only to eat, but to call Ed. What is he doing? With whom? I need to get myself together for me. And God, if I come to know Him that way. I want to be able to say to a man I'm involved with, "go ahead and do what you want." I want to be able to function alone.

Enormous anger again. I yelled at my animals.

Suddenly the compulsion was gone, as simply as if a light switch had been pressed. I don't know why it happened.

I told Ruth about Ed. She said, "You know how psychiatrists don't give advice — tell you what to do?"

"Yeah."

"Well, sponsors do. Don't see him."

"Why not?"

"You don't have enough abstinence or program behind you. Take it slower."

(73)

In state of binge or kill myself. Ed phoned to say he feels he'd better not see me so much, maybe not talk together so much.

Shit. I'll eat. No, I won't. He's not worth blowing my abstinence.

If I cried, I'd cry. One analyst said that was in itself an improvement in my psyche — at least to know I'd be crying, if I cried.

Ruth, you said to write, that there's always a reason for feeling lousy.

The reason I want to eat is because a light bulb went out today and now Ed won't be here to fix it. Just write on, she says.

I'll call Ed and see if he's there. That way I can tell him I agree we'd better not talk.

I must not call Ed. Or anyone. I need to be self-sufficient.
Nobody will ever love me.

Eating never really stopped craziness. Or did it?

When can I stop writing?

If I get up now and go out and binge, I can begin
the agony all over again. Winchells, Baskin-Robbins, cake
and vanilla ice cream. Begin it all over again, this unceasing, agonizing eating, pleasant for a few days, excruciating
agony for a month. The horror at school. Lane Bryant.

Tonight is the first time I have believed the disease
is totally psychological. It may be true that physically
there's no turn-off button but the turn-on button is totally
psychological.

It seems a reasonable idea to die. All that I have going
against this idea is being alive. The only conclusive evidence I have of anything is that life wants to go on living.
I want to kill myself rather than gain the weight back
or keep going through nights like this, but over and over
again I return to the thought that what seems to be such
a reasonable idea — to be dead — must have something
wrong at the root of it, for everywhere about me flowers
bloom and giggling children cannot be quieted by sternest
admonitions.

(74)

Dream. Eating at school. Ladyfingers. Doing it before
I knew. All teachers there. Go to my room desperate.
Remember what Ruth said to a girl who had broken
her abstinence: You haven't lost it, start over. But I am
in a trapped state of despair. Eating in classroom, unable
to relate to children. Forcing myself to think of lessons.
When I get to the room someone else is teaching the
children to read.

Woke. *I am not my body, but I am my behavior.*

I remember going to lunch last year the first day. I
ordered the biggest omelette, though I was stuffed already.

Please, Higher Power out there, please take me to lunch on Monday.

(75)

Made it through a P.T.A. lunch. Everybody continues to be thrilled by my weight loss. They are eager to hear the method. I try to explain that OA is only for compulsive overeaters. They think they are compulsive overeaters. Everybody in America thinks she's a compulsive overeater.

(76)

Theory of Special Occasions for Hugging

Hugging is done only on returns from long trips or long farewells. Kiss and hug goodnight normal until maybe five or six years old. Our society fucks up hugging. Just about none unless death, or wedding, or a birth. It averages out to about two hugs a year over a lifetime. When I lived in Turkey I remember men holding hands, men embracing, women always arm in arm. Doesn't seem to make a difference in national life, but it does in personal life, I'll bet. In Re-Eval you hug strangers you've no feeling for — like that in lots of encounter stuff. Phony hugging is worse than no hugging. We do have a lot of phony hugging everywhere we go. I'm not counting any of that in my averaging. In OA we get to want to hug people. Or so they tell me.

Sexual hugging is different. We all know that affection is sex, though not always present and certainly not the determining factor in sexual activity in America (deodorants and good cups of coffee are the determining factors), is definitely permissible.

Anything with orgasm as intent is okay in this culture.

(77)

Conversation at Work

"Karen, did you read *Manchild in a Promised Land?*"
"No, I haven't."
"Autobiography of Malcolm X?"
"Part of it. Too depressing to go on."
"What do you read? I've always thought of you as a reader, intelligent."
"Books about religion, or religious books, both of those."
"Religion???" (My co-worker is stopped dead, speechless; if I had said I was doing research into the growths of various seeds of opium, it would have gone over better.)
"But, Karen, that's irrelevant."
"What?"
"Religion."
"Not to me."
"Oh, come on, in today's world religion is out."
"Why don't we just not talk?"
"But you've got a high I.Q."
"Did you ever read anything about Martin Luther King's I.Q.?"
"Oh, come on. King was a fighter. A man for his people. His religion was just a tool to get him his people."
"Go away."
"Ministers are the lowest I.Q. group of the nation."
"Based on what?"
"Observation. All you need to do is look."
"Go away, please. Go read your relevant books, and show me how you change the world."
"While you pray?"
"If I want to, I'll even pray."
I have a dream that "one day every valley shall be exalted, and every mountain and hill shall be made low,

the crooked shall be made straight and the rough places plain, and the glory of the Lord shall be revealed. . ." (Isaiah 40:3-4).

I have defended the faith, and I feel better, but crushed. What in hell do you do with the bigots? Especially when there's all that they say always running through your own brain, of your own making. There's always an awful line of reasoning which can drop you off at the spot at which you must conclude that God, the ultimate stork, dropped them off.

And then, of course, there's always the lettuce girl, pitching away, losing weight. Yesterday God gave her a parking place at The Farmer's Market.

She is radiant and jubilant, saved and sincere; the pounds are falling away from her.

Five million children die of starvation, and God, the highest power, picks her lettuce.

Maybe he's like me. Just tackle the solvable problems.

God gave someone else four baseball tickets to a Dodgers Series game. No one on earth could have swung that deal. The man who goes to baseball games is now thin. Pity. God has the peanut concession too.

And this is the place I need to be to be saved?

God doesn't play dice with the universe.

— Albert Einstein

God doesn't pick lettuce heads.

— Karen R.

(78)

Me pitching.

"Hi, my name is Karen. I'm a compulsive overeater. When I first got here I thought that the Serenity Prayer, when it said, accept the things you cannot change . . .

that part, I locked into, thinking I had to learn acceptance. I thought I could change nothing. In my head, bent through years of psychiatry to fight depression, my problems were so unconscious that I came to think nothing could change. The program, and listening to all of you, has just hit me with the sane idea that Steps Six and Seven make possible a lot of change. I have some character defects to work on. When I'm jealous I always feel I am guilty only of picking relationships which make me feel jealousy. Like my unconscious programs me for jealousy by picking a man to have an affair with who is already taken. Or who is a looker after all other women. Maybe that is my unconscious doing it, but the jealousy and possessiveness — define them as character defects, which by God they are although never before was I bright enough to think of them as such, and I am responsible to myself and to others (all of OA) to change the defects. My defects are not immutably fixed, like astrological designations. I manipulate; I'm jealous and possessive; I'm filled with cowardice and an unwillingness to brave pain.

"These are not forces in the natural and unnatural world attacking me. I'll attack back. I'll work the Steps of the program. Thank you."

Later. Is this a spiritual awakening? Maybe. I wonder how long it lasts. Ed's has since he turned his will and his alcoholism and his life over to God. Many years. Ruth too. Many, many. No refined carbohydrates.

Neatly summarized this means:

1. If I am jealous, I lose.
2. If I am possessive, I lose.
3. If I am afraid, I lose.

I want to win, to grow, and to change. Tonight was uncomfortable but I'm getting through it, without eating and without depression.

(79)

Ruth and I saw *Earthquake,* one of those crummy movies that I love passionately. Thought about it a lot later, about quakes and that kind of death. I see that you can lose all belief and yet if you believe that the world is made valid by your own individual courage or invalid by your lack of courage, then you have a continual, sensible reason to go on and can go on until there is no longer a you to go on. The hope of courage never dies; cowardly act upon cowardly act does not deny the chance that at the end, at the propitious time, you will come through for yourself. That is enough to keep a man going.

(80)

I will never break my abstinence. This is my chosen way of life. I weigh 150. The holidays do not frighten me.

(81)

Thanksgiving Day
It was just one piece of apple pie and one scoop of chocolate ice cream. And for no discernible reason.
It was there and I was there. In the company of normies. One split second of forgetting who I am and what I am.

(82)

The plunge is dizzying. I'm falling so fast I can't look up or down and in front of me is pitch dark.

Part Four

Turning It Over

One bite is too many — a thousand, not enough.
— Overeaters Anonymous

A spiritual quest is only possible if something has happened to you without your knowing. It may be love, it may be in music, it may be in nature, it may be in friendship. It may be in any communion. Something has happened to you that has been a source of bliss and it is now just a remembering, a memory. It may not even be a conscious memory; it may be unconscious. It may be waiting like a seed somewhere deep within you. This seed will become the source of a quest, and you will go on searching for something that you do not know. What are you searching for? You do not know. But still, somewhere, even unknown to you, some experience, some blissful moment has become part and parcel of your mind. It has become a seed, and now that seed is working its way through, and you are in quest of something which you cannot name, which you cannot explain.

— Bhagwan Shree Rajneesh,
Meditation: The Art of Ecstacy

The pain that one feels at having claimed one's own identity is enormous.

— Norene Harris, conversation, 1976

Eternal vigilance is the price of abstinence.

— me

Made a decision to turn my will and my life over to the care of God as I understood him

— God, please help me?
— Will you do Step Three with me?
— Well, I mean . . .
Well, what do you mean?
— Can I do it a little?
— Do you want a little or a lot of help?
— You mean I can bargain?
— No.
and He went away.

Dream. It was a task to be of the group. I had to go into this big arena room to overcome a fear. I didn't know what my task in the big arena would be. I hesitated, tried to find a way to know what I had to do before I was in there trying to do it. Maybe take LSD, I thought. The leader said to me, "Unless you go, you will never know what the task is."

I realize it was a case of "For whosoever will save his life shall lose it and whosoever will lose his life for my sake shall find it."

I went. There were only hurdles I needed to jump over. If I jumped I might break a leg, but that would be the worst of it. It was an initiation rite of a cult of consciousness.

(2)

I have a glimpse of how you're supposed to do Step Three. I've gotten that close. Haven't done it yet but I see how. Maybe. You just do it. Step Three is a little like going down Dead Man's Hill in Prospect Park, with snow only on about half the slope and rocks jutting everywhere uncovered. With that in front of your eyes, you just do it. There is a space between the top of the hill and just below the top. It is in that space that you have suddenly made the leap.

(3)

Faith is a place in your head that concerns itself with your ability or inability to act in a certain way. Faith is a way of acting, a way also of drawing courage from a purer source than that of ego. Faith is not something one gets, though you may have gone out to get it: it is a territory to be achieved.

(4)

What am I doing wrong? I go to meetings. "Bring the body and the mind will follow. . . . Keep coming back. . . . Listen, listen, listen."

I need Step One. But, after all this time, what do they think of my needing so much more help. I can't ask for help all the time, every day, day after day. No, I can't ask again. I'll just eat my way back to 200 pounds.

I'll help you work your program but damned if I'll

repeat the course myself. I'm the kid who skipped grades and beat the high school system and the college dungeons by years. Always way ahead. You want me to repeat the course.

No.

(5)

"Hi, my name is Larry. I'm a compulsive overeater, and your leader for tonight. I came in at 350 plus. It was probably more. I have been maintaining 125 for over a year now. At the beginning I had trouble getting the abstinence, but once I got it, the abstinence itself has held me up and saved me. I didn't know anything about myself or the world out there for an entire lifetime. I am only beginning to see myself, beginning to know a truth that would have been unacceptable to me. I did not accept reality and I did not know myself. There really isn't any difference between losing 250 pounds or 50 pounds, once you've lost them, but living with them is different. It's the degree of hiding that has gone on in your lifetime. The heavier you are the more you can hide. My own theory is that how much fat you have on you is directly related to how much of your unconscious you have not dealt in any way with. Through my sponsors I started to get up all the feelings that made me eat. And they are still coming up, I can tell you that. It's hard to share the program because it's hard to reproduce the crying I did. Man to man, I cried. And got held. And lost weight. You shouldn't get the medals for the weight loss but for the years of struggle. The yoyo years, the obsession always there.

"A lot of people identify with being told they're angry. I identified with fear. I never went out so I was afraid of everything beyond my kitchen and my mom's help-fulness in my life. . . .

"There came a time when I knew a split second in which I gave it all up to God. And the fears are gone. And the abstinence remains. . . ."

(6)

I really heard Larry about the crying. I know I need to learn to cry — that crying changes things for a woman, that it is not just giving in to self-pity and weakness.

I talked to my "normie" friend, Roberta, today.

"Karen, I've been eating and eating and eating. I can't stop. You must promise not to tell anyone if I tell you how much I weigh."

"Okay, Roberta, I promise."

"No one, not even J."

"No one, not even J." (I know that a week ago she weighed some perfect weight or other, a great figure, so I know whatever is coming at me isn't going to be easy to take, but I do not know how to stop its coming.)

"I weigh 130 pounds! I've gained 3 pounds in a week. I look grotesque. I wouldn't tell anybody but you."

"Glad you told me, Roberta. Really glad you could share."

I get off the phone as fast as I can. It is easier to control the crying impulse when not engaged in conversation.

I remember how I stopped crying.

I was five, playing in a playground near old Ebbets Field. We lived a few blocks away. My mother sat near by on a bench talking with the other mothers whose children were playing. I came down hard off the slide, fell forward onto my knees, and when I looked at one knee which was paining me, I saw the blood oozing out. I wanted to cry then, but I felt I should first get to my mother. I limped over. Once I got there, it was okay to cry.

"I wanna go home."

"Oh, you fell."

She got up, gathered up my balls and a jacket, and we started walking home. She had tried to stop the blood with tissues and it was a little better, but it was still bleeding.

It was still bleeding. My knee.

And she stopped on the street to talk to a friend.

While I stood there and bled. And I cried.

She talked to her friend until she had talked enough. By then I had decided never to let her see me cry again.

Looking back, I know that what is a heavy flow of blood to a five-year-old may be a scratch with no danger attached. But she had miffed her chance to take care of me. She would not get another.

Had I been a compulsive eater then, I would no doubt have eaten up all the oatmeal and graham crackers in Brooklyn.

In OA and AA they say that "Resentment is the number one killer." Resentments make you eat, drink, help form the basis of the compulsions that besiege the world.

Arnie Stone used to make me cry. He'd wait for me after school and twist my arm behind my back until I begged him to stop. I cried then and he'd stop. Arnie Stone twisted my arm for months. And I never went home by another route. Toward the end I learned not to cry, even from the pain. And then he dropped me.

In the movies I cry. Or reading. If you say to me "Mother, child, child dies," I sob. But only in a movie, only with a book. In real life I curse God and move away as fast as I can.

I have begun to recognize the techniques I use to prevent my crying. I think if I can see what I do, maybe I'll be able to change back into the five-year-old, have a good cry and ever after cry when I'm hurt — like people.

How do I do it? When I feel it coming at me, when the insult, or the tragic news, is coming in at me, I mentally leave. A man once told me that in making love, in order not to have an orgasm too quickly, he thought about other things (like picking up your suit at the cleaners — he wasn't a romantic at heart). I think that's what I do. I go to pick up my suit at the cleaners and I don't cry.

(7)

"Joyce, everybody's watching me eat again."

"Karen, they just feel bad for you."

"No, they don't. Zena's gloating."

"That's true."

"It's hopeless."

"You told me OA says that if you go to meetings, there's no such thing as a hopeless case. Is that true?"

"So they say."

"Are you going to meetings?"

"Yes."

"So. Check out your classroom for any planted eclairs and in you go."

(8)

Ah, yes, Ed is divorcing his wife and running about with an OA girl. Ah, yes.

(9)

Ruth: I can't stand the self-pity stages, Karen. The self-pity of the compulsive overeater is the hardest character defect we have to overcome.

Karen: But, Ruth . . .

Ruth: You're going to have to grow up. You have a disease, other people have diseases — enough already. You have to stop the eating, period. I don't care if James Caan offers you a drink. On second thought, I'll give you a dispensation. If James Caan offers you a drink you can have it.

Karen: Sorry, but I never drink, under any circumstances.

(10)

A. says that old addicts eventually give up going out to get the stuff. They're too worn out. There's nothing left of them to even hype up. The spirit is gone. When is the spirit gone irretrievably? Does anyone go among derelicts to pass out God and solace? I'm an age of derelicts.

(11)

Original Existentialist Position Paper:
You can't have your cake and eat it too.

(12)

I have started to do exactly what Ruth tells me, simply because she tells me. No arguments from me. I am praying all the time. I am waking up into the Shema, I do the Lord's Prayer, and the Twenty-third Psalm all the way to work and, whenever possible, even there. I keep the words, "Not my will, but Thy will," going through my head. I offer myself to God, to build with and to do with what He wants. Nevertheless, I eat all the time. Cereal at home, stop at McDonald's, recess, lunch, on the drive home from school.

Over and over, Ruth's voice saying, "You will get your abstinence back, Karen. You will get your abstinence back. In God's time."

(13)

Intellectuals in particular still have the illusion
that they can apply standard logic in an attempt
to understand reality.
— Marilyn Ferguson, *The Aquarian Conspiracy*

The question of change, the split second of change in
belief systems. That is the most enticing autobiographical
question I know. What makes it happen?

The split second between the bud and the rose
is known only to those who become roses.
                                        — Reshad Feild

(14)

A week later
Hurrah, I have two days of abstinence. I have had
to stay in the house, home from school, to get it. I gave
Rhoda my car keys and asked her if I could phone in
my food to her for a few days. She said okay.

(15)

Oh damn. At loose again. A devouring animal set onto
the freeway. Since I left Joyce, I have driven all over
town looking for pumpkin pie and cheesecake and ice
cream. I brought it all home. I am eating as I write.
Annie thinks Christmas has come again.
Why? Because I met a new man at Joyce's, and when
I refused a drink — because one drink and I forget all
thought of abstaining (alcohol is basically sugar, they tell
me) — and he insisted, I took the drink. If only I could
have gotten the words "hypoglycemic" or "alcoholic" out
of my mouth. (An alcoholic has status.) I just stood there

and knew I could never say "compulsive overeater" to any faintly eligible man. The words would not come out of my mouth. I drank the proffered drink, which had crème de cacao in it, and laughed and chatted and certainly had no food problems. Until I left for the drive home.

I am an addict. I must refuse to go to dinners, especially in the holiday season. I'm doing it all over again. The guilt, the throwing up, the dog shitting all over from eating pie, cake, and all of this.

I am an addict in a dark room in a movie nobody sees but once.

The worst thing in the world is eating. The next worst thing is not eating.

I've tried hard enough to go on living and I haven't made it.

(16)

The days of eating wear on. It has been two weeks. I have already gained 15 pounds.

I must stop. It is true what they say in meetings: the food doesn't work for you any more. I called Ruth and was told: "You can choose to binge or go through whatever it is you have to go through. Of course it takes courage to go through whatever it is ... it's easier to binge." So I went out and binged and thought, with the delicious first bite, there now, doesn't this taste good? So much better than courage.

But driving home again, miserable, yet it occurred to me that even in this myriad surfeiting, life is grand (not grand like nice, but on a sweeping scale grand). Tonight it rains from Winchells to Baskin and a splendor is shining through.

(17)

Get this now. Somewhere during the days of this binge

I called Bullocks to get two new sheets in denim blue. And when the lady said they were out of them, I said, "Oh," in such a sad tone because I couldn't get my patchy denim blues that my tone got Mrs. Walker at the other end in Bullocks to say she'd see if they could order them. There is a madness that escapes the mind's analysis. That is not true of all madness. But it is true of mine — witness denim blues.

How could anybody who orders denim blues in the midst of a death-defying binge while doing the triple not get well? I must come out of this. I expect to stop bingeing and I expect to be thin and to have energy return.

T. told me that she always knew she'd grow up to be an alcoholic. When the other kids would talk about what they wanted to be, she'd say something like a nurse, but she knew she'd be an alcoholic.

As a kid, I used to have a vision come upon me sometimes in the movies of being very down and then being saved. I'll bet being saved is a universal fantasy of some sort or other. That's all humanity may have going for it, when you really think about it, the intuition that we need to be saved.

(18)

Weak again today. Please, no more. Called Ruth. I started my usual debate. She said, "Aren't you sick to death of the whys physical and the whys mental? Just don't eat."

We've all about had it with me, I think.

Ms. Hepburn is trying to get my tootsie roll.

(19)

Pray, they all say.

(20)

"Hi, my name is Laura and I'm an abstaining, grateful compulsive overeater ... All who have maintained have made the religious psychic change. There are a few AA's and OA's I know who lost the weight without the change and are keeping sober, clean, and thin, but they aren't people anybody wants to be with. It's just that simple. Surrender is the key. You throw in the last towel. I couldn't and I couldn't and I did and then I said to my sponsor, 'You mean that's all there is to it?' 'Yes,' she said. 'You had to make the decision. Nobody else could do it for you, you had to do it for yourself.'"

(21)

Don't I know that's the key? I just don't have the right towels. How many surrenders do there have to be, by the way?

Is it a *koan?*

(22)

Overheard at Marathon: "As I walk with God I stop running, and as I stop running I can face myself."

(23)

"Ruth, I'm not going to make it through the night."

"Come over here. You can sleep on the couch."

"But Al ..."

"He's used to it. Remember, he's an alcoholic. Just a little bit more Twelfth Step work as far as he's concerned."

"If I leave this house, I'll eat."

"Fine, we'll talk until you can get here without eating."

Long pause.

"Okay, Ruth. I'll get there without eating."

"Come, we're watching TV. You might even enjoy yourself."

Even driving from Beverly Hills to Hollywood is a challenge filled with junk food stations along the way. But how can I not make it? I mean she's offering me her house — how can I let her down? Banana split, chocolate-covered bear claw — I even think of picking up some spaghetti to bring over. My mother says you should never visit anybody without bringing them something.

I make it there. I am surprised to realize I have never been there before. I see that her telephone is blue. It matches the color tones of her living room. Everything in her house is comfortable, lived in.

I have met her husband before. He is short and well built, nearly bald, handsome and strong. Hard to picture him drunk.

"Hi," he says. "Good to see you."

"I hope I'm not intruding."

"Just don't take the first drink, that's all."

We all laugh.

We are watching TV and the pain comes back, the undefinable pain that is like breakers at the beach thrashing against my skull in its desire to break through some barrier in my skull, also undefinable. The compulsion returns and I think I will get up and leave. I hang in, watching police and car chases, and plots I doubt I could follow even when not obsessed.

After a while, Alan excuses himself and leaves us. Ruth, her face a little lined, a little tired, yet her eyes as full of light as ever, turns to me. "How you doing?"

"Oh, fine."

"Karen, 'oh, fine' won't do. Where are you in your head?"

"I don't know." I do know, though. In my head, I

am frightened, sad, angry, hurting. I try to say as much to Ruth.

"Why the anger?"

"I don't know."

"You do. It just doesn't come out easily."

"But I don't know why I'm angry. Or at what."

"Okay, forget that. It doesn't matter anyway, the damn whys."

She gets up and goes to a closet and brings me linens for the couch. Together we make up my sleeping quarters.

"Are you safe, Karen? Can I go to bed?"

Oh, my God. Is she going to leave me?

"Well," I say.

We're upstairs. I awaken instantly mobilized if I hear a refrigerator door open, remember that.

I know she has the real stuff in this refrigerator for the thin one. I try to laugh, but will I make it through the night?

"Give us a hug goodnight," she says.

I draw back, pushing into the couch.

She laughs. "It's time you learned that hugs are relevant."

She puts her arms around me and hugs me. I burst into tears. Just like that. I cry and cry and cry. She doesn't say a word. Goes for Kleenex, comes back, and stays with me. I cry for at least fifteen minutes. I become conscious of my crying and embarrassed and guilty that I am keeping Ruth up. Between nose blowings I try to say that.

"Okay," she says. "I'll go to sleep. Are you going to be all right?"

I knew I would be. I smiled. "I never cry," I say.

"I know," she says.

I sleep through the night. The refrigerator goes unmolested.

(24)

If I am not for myself
Who will be for me?
And if I am only for myself
Who am I?
And if not now, when?

— Reb Hillel

(25)

Something incredible just happened tonight. I was just going through it over and over again and again. I won't go to the meeting. I'll eat. No, I won't eat, I'll go to the meeting; no, I'll stay home and read. I'll call my sponsor but I won't eat. I will eat. I want to eat. Why shouldn't I eat? Just this once?

And the weariness at last was ultimate. I asked, finally, in surrender, that inexplicable state of mind, state of being, "God, please take it away, just stop all this about the food, I mean it, I've had it, please take it away." My words are almost gone already. What was it I actually said? I know that it was where I was in my spirit, when I said it, not what I said. I turned it over. And God took it away.

Yea, verily.

(26)

Yet the obsession comes back. Do I have to go through it all again? Today?

(27)

Last night at the meeting, I heard: "Yesterday I was

a compulsive overeater, today I am a compulsive over-eater, but by the grace of God, just for today, just for this moment, I have been relieved of the obsession — just for this moment."

Why not permanent relief? I asked Faye's sponsor Frank and was told that God demands each man be reborn each day. I understood when I was walking with Frank and he said, "Why should we need more than this day? To see the simple day out there." He made it glisten.

(28)

A prayer finally locks into the place of my brain. Onto my tongue. It is one I have said so many times, but suddenly when I say it: "God relieve me of the bondage of self so that I may better do Thy will," something is changing within me. Thy will, not my will.

Everything clicks. It is irrational, no doubt about it — but that, being that, aside — I see that *everything is God's Will.* I cannot defend or think about free will.

Therefore, whether I eat or not is not going to be a question of my will, or God's helping me to do my will. When I've been out there gobbling and squawking, that has been God's will. For some reason.

I say the prayer over and over and over again, for days.

(29)

Today was the fifth day of the prayer. I have started to abstain.

Sixth, seventh, eighth. Abstaining. Beginning to feel the sugar go out of me. Physically barely making it through a day, then coming home and sleeping a lot. But whenever awake, the prayer.

(30)

It's back. The obsession. I must fight it through. God, please relieve me of this compulsion to binge. If it be Thy will, Lord, relieve me of the compulsion to binge.

I am bundled in God's world. If I eat tonight, it is God's will. But I will keep asking God to relieve me of the obsession. If I am not relieved of the obsession, then it is God's will that I eat. I cannot hang myself any more on the issue of my eating. A marble doesn't get moved in the marble jar without the universe's being affected. Lord, please relieve me of this obsession.

It looks like I'm going to eat. I go out for banana cake with white frosting. I drive to the Gourmet Shop in the Gulch. Through the door. Second door among see through doors. Second section. Middle row. No banana cake.

I am tempted to think that God made it this way for me on purpose, but I am not that mushy-headed yet. I say to myself, Hollywood Ranch Market will have it. I'll get it, being it's defrosting, and get to Baskin-Robbins before 10:30.

I go in through the seedy crowd, past the ice cream, the cookies, and by now I am saying, "God, please relieve me of this obsession if it be Thy will ..." I must have my banana cake. I continue my prayer as I muck my hand about in the freezing cold aluminum-encrusted cardboard-covered sets of Sara Lee's stuff. No banana cake.

I think Sara Lee must have flipped out. Maybe she's phasing it out. I am continuing my prayer. This time I do think maybe it is a gift from God. But I consider cream cheesecake, and every other item. I am praying. Don't let anybody say that you can't do or think two things at the same time — you sure as hell can. Also a voice saying, "Of course you'll eat, of course you'll eat.

God's will is a lot of crap. You're just working for a rationalization of why you must go on eating. Bullshit."

Also playing in this tape deck is a number dealing with how God affects the mighty Sara Lee industry. The phone rings at Sara Lee. She answers herself.
— Yes.
— No banana cake anywhere in Los Angeles on October 14.
— Again? We did this last week in Anaheim.
Grumbling is heard through the factory.
The voice out of the whirlwind speaks again: "Who are you to say to me, again? Yes. Again.
He hangs up.
The workers set about their task.
Vibrations are felt in Nicaragua.
Suddenly all of the orchestration ceases. I am laughing. I am breathing. The obsession is gone.
I feel that I am walking in a safe place. I comprehend that even if I had eaten it would have been God's will.
I hope that I will remember the feeling and the learning.
I drive home, call Ruth, and tell it all to her.
"Yes," she says. "Yes."

(31)

Five days later

From the incident, the turning it over in the frozen-food-department experience, my abstinence has sprung.

(32)

Jesus, I'm turning into an evangelist. I never wanted to be an evangelist. Maybe I always wanted to be an evangelist. Some things from my childhood come back to me. Once, I remember — I must have been six or so — standing in my bedroom, which looked out over the backyard and the clotheslines, and as I turned from the window, I felt a change in the room — as if it were being filled with more than the light coming in. I looked at the bed, and the bureau, and again outside, and everything was changed. I remember thinking, God is all of this stuff. And God is me. It suddenly frightened me, and I went into the living room. My parents were watching TV, and everything in that room was the same as ever. There were no words I could think of to tell them what had happened to me, so I sat down and watched the show with them. That made them feel good — I always remember them saying, "All you do is shut yourself up in that room."

And I remember, years later, a similar experience.

It was winter. I was jumping on snow packed along the edges of the street, packed so high one could imagine it a long series of igloos — jumping in exultation under the lamplight alone on the snow, freezing, out beyond my bedtime, a disobedient child — and there again, a presence that made the place more than it was.

Again, I described it to no one.

(33)

I remind myself of a kid I had in the fourth grade, early in my teaching career. She still hadn't been able to comprehend that five plus seven not only equals twelve, but that seven plus five also equals twelve, and for good reasons. I tried every way available — flannel boards, magic slates, coins, etc. But I never did feel I'd gotten it across. Never even approached three plus two plus three equals five plus three.

She went on to the fifth grade, a very sweet and diligent girl. She came in very excited after a few weeks with Miss Levine across the hall and said, "Miss R., Miss R., look, I want to show you something: Three plus two equals five, and it's the same as two plus three equals five."

"That's fantastic, Anita, fantastic."

I mean I wasn't one to say, I told you so. And then she said, nicely, but with some tinge of resentment, "Miss R., why didn't you ever tell me that?"

(34)

My abstinence continues. I get to lead a meeting.

"Hi, my name is Karen, and I'm a compulsive overeater. It has taken me almost a year to realize that in a twelve-step program the numbers go from one to twelve. You can't keep abstaining indefinitely only by admitting you're powerless and grabbing for restored sanity while you debate with God over the question of where His will begins and yours leaves off.

"Don't think I don't still catch myself thinking: if I do it right, then can I eat? The answer is No. My life depends on my answering no every day one day at a time.

"If, on the program, you are able to listen well enough, there's the hope a change will occur in you that will have the question itself drop out of your mind. You cannot remove the question, the desire to eat, so don't even try. Work a program one day at a time. If the question and desire are to be removed, only God can remove them. In His time.

"You will have to continue to abstain the pain if that is the only way you can abstain. It hurts less to hurt from not eating than to hurt from eating. But I don't want to kid you. It hurts incessantly and hard either way. But one way leads to a psychic change, a life lived in a new state of consciousness.

"My sponsor told me, Karen, the only way you can learn more about yourself is by beating out the attacking compulsion. This has continued to be true on this program.

"A few weeks ago I was at a conference called Mind

as Healer, Mind as Slayer and heard Stephanie Simonton talk about her work with cancer patients in the terminal part of their illnesses. She was a speaker of rare beauty and the entire audience was hushed, so it was clear that everybody in the room was involved. Suddenly I had a great compulsion to eat — quick, I must get out, must eat. And because I no longer follow that order when it crosses my mind, I asked myself, how could I flip out of what she was saying, when I'd been listening so intently? And I tucked back in and realized that most of the audience was crying. I listened. She had been talking about the last moments and thoughts of a dying man — I could, so to speak, listen backwards and get that. And I saw that I had, without even consciously doing it, seen ahead to what would have been exposing myself to pain, and had blocked the pain with the obsession, without any conscious knowledge. Had I gotten up and gone out to eat, I would not have realized how thorough my protective mechanism is. So thorough it even keeps me from knowing what particular pain I'm missing.

"Which would be all well and good except it means you're missing life too. But I have begun to cry and will cry some more, and so will miss less life.

"I have been then, a compendium of anger, fear, grief, and faithlessness. And it has taken the strength of a million meals to keep it all down and then the strength of a million friends to know that God can only get through when you aren't using all your energies to repress feelings.

"You have probably already noticed that I am the type who tries, almost on a daily basis and in every pitch, to summarize my life and get something out of it." (I never could understand someone auditing a class in college — I mean if you didn't get the credits, then what were you there for?) "I still do this, but I have begun to see, thanks to my disease and looking for surcease from it, that this attitude is pretty sick in itself. We really have very little to do with choosing the courses we will take. And auditing is fine.

"I'm supposedly up here to share with you my experience, strength, and hope. I've been backlogging the experience and I have a little strength now and a lot of hope. The hope is that if I continue to let go of the compulsion for a bit and work my Twelve Steps I will be able to abstain from compulsive overeating one day at a time for at least twenty-four hours. Thank you."

(35)

Suddenly I have a lot to say. I feel I have got somewhere. I have again six weeks of abstinence. I had it once before. But something is different this time. I see the whole thing now as working on my inside. Like you only get this tiny little bit of consciousness-unconsciousness which is to be all your own — your private store for your very own hang-ups and fuck-ups. It's very small, this space, takes up hardly the neurons of the rest of your unconscious-consciousness, but it will be, when you are finished, your contribution to eternity. It's all a mystery still, but I am certain that that tiny space, surrounded by God, but not of God, that tiny space in your head is what you get to give to God — to prepare and to handle and to grieve through until you feel the ecstasy of all the outside of it and all that which you can bring inside.

Ecstasy spreads then, wildfire through the neurons, and God permeates and sings — it is the axon of all time.

Now I see life as a call. I understand for the first time about Prometheus and the flame, the risks he took, the glamor of it and the danger. I see the fireball in the heavens and think it is my soul that is the fireball, my soul that is the heavens. All this information was left out of the classrooms and the study halls, but I did learn that "my soul is a tattered and a paltry thing." So that fireball cannot be my soul. This brick-orange-burning reddening ball must be *our* soul — the soul that all of us breathe in and out. The soul that all of us are traveling within and on, and through.

(36)

I have stopped counting days. I am disciplined again. I try to work my program one day at a time.

I've always had imaginary people asking me questions like: Are you happy? Are you cured? Etc. Now I answer. It's a nice day out there, and in any one day I'm going to be suicidal and jubilant, fat and thin, terrified and brave.

But, next week, on our Bicentennial Day, when we let fly the two-hundred balloons and cheer on the children in their costumes and do indeed glory in our freedom here in this country, I feel good in my freedom. Tentative though it, like all freedom, is, I have a feeling (as long as I do what I'm told each twenty-four hours between now and then) that I'll still have mine.

I want it. When I'm offered the big, beautiful cake, with the lovely flag and candles and "Happy Birthday" on it, I want to be able to say: "No, thank you. I'm not eating anything red, white, or blue today."

(37)

Come, come, whoever you are,
Wanderer, worshipper, lover of leaving,
It doesn't matter.

Ours is not a caravan of despair.
Come, even if you have broken your vow a thousand
times.
Come, yet again, come, come.

— Mevlana Jelalu'ddin Rumi

The way is sacred; you cannot own it.

Acknowledgements

Basic Books, Inc., for permission to quote from *Eating Disorders; Obesity, Anorexia Nervosa, and the Person Within*, by Hilde Bruch, M.D. © 1973 by Basic Books, Inc., New York.

Health Science, for permission to quote from *The Miracle of Fasting*, by Paul Bragg. © by Health Science, Santa Barbara, California.

Princeton University Press, for permission to quote from *I Ching*, by Richard Wilhelm, rendered into English by Cary Baynes, © 1950, 1967, renewed 1977, by Princeton University Press, Bollingen Series, Princeton, New Jersey.

Anchor Books, for permission to quote from *The Interior Castle*, from *The Complete Works of St. Theresa of Avila*, translated by E. Allison Peers, from the *Critical Edition of P. Silverio-De Sainte Theresa, C.D.*, © 1972 by Sheed & Ward, New York.

Bhagwan Shree Rajneesh, for permission to quote from *Meditation: The Art of Ecstasy*, by Bhagwan Shree Rajneesh (Harper & Row, Publishers, Harper Colophon Books), © 1976 by Rajneesh Foundation, by permission of Harper & Row, Publishers, Inc.

Shambhala Publications, Inc., for permission to quote from *Cutting Through Spiritual Materialism*, by Chogyam Trungpa, © 1975 Shambhala Publications, Inc., Boulder, Colorado.

HERE IS YOUR CHANCE TO ORDER SOME OF OUR BEST

HISTORICAL ROMANCES

BY SOME OF YOUR FAVORITE AUTHORS

____ **DARK WINDS** — Virginia Coffman
Their fiery passion unleashed a tempest of . . . DARK
WINDS. 7701-0405-3/$3.95

____ **KISS OF GOLD** — Samantha Harte
First he taught her to live . . . then he taught her to love.
7701-0529-7/$3.50

____ **MISTRESS OF MOON HILL** — Jill Downie
From the ashes of her heart, he kindled a new flame.
7701-0424-X/$3.95

____ **SWEET WHISPERS** — Samantha Harte
She struggled with her dark past in the hope of a new love.
7701-0496-7/$3.50

____ **THE WIND & THE SEA** — Marsha Canham
Passion and intrigue on the high seas. 7701-0415-0/$3.95

____ **TIME TO LOVE** — Helen McCullough
Love triumphs in a desperate time. 7701-0560-2/$3.95

Prices subject to change without notice

- -

BOOKS BY MAIL

320 Steelcase Rd. E.   210 5th Ave., 7th Floor
Markham, Ont., L3R 2M1   New York, N.Y. 10010

Please send me the books I have checked above. I am enclosing a total of $_____ (Please add 1.00 for one book and
50 cents for each additional book.) My cheque or money order
is enclosed. (No cash or C.O.D.'s please.)

Name _____

Address _____ Apt. _____

City _____

Prov./State _____ P.C./Zip _____

(HIS/ROM)

BESTSELLING
SELF-HELP TITLES

from
PaperJacks

____**BOUNCING BACK** — Andrew J. DuBrin Ph.D.
                                         7701-03189/$2.95
How to handle setbacks in your work and personal
life.

____**CRY ANGER** — Jack Birnbaum M.D.   7701-04428/$3.50
A common-sense do-it-yourself approach to fighting
the biggest epidemic of our times — DEPRESSION.

____**IN THE CENTER OF THE NIGHT** — Jayne Blankenship
                                         7701-04002/$3.95
A story of survival against the despair of her
husband's death, and the gradual healing of herself
and, in the process, others.

____**WHAT DID I DO WRONG?** — Lynn Caine 7701-04185/$3.95
Mothering and guilt.

Prices subject to change without notice

BOOKS BY MAIL

320 Steelcase Rd. E.   210 5th Ave., 7th Floor
Markham, Ont., L3R 2M1   New York, N.Y. 10010

Please send me the books I have checked above. I am
enclosing a total of $_____ (Please add 1.00 for
one book and 50 cents for each additional book.) My
cheque or money order is enclosed. (No cash or
C.O.D.'s please.)

Name _____

Address _____ Apt. _____

City _____

Prov./State _____ P.C./Zip _____

                                              (SH/2)

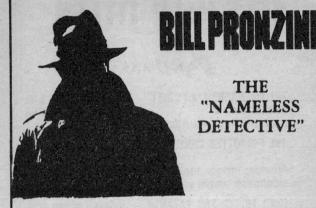

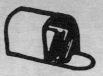

FREE!!
BOOKS BY MAIL
CATALOGUE

BOOKS BY MAIL will share with you our current bestselling books as well as hard to find specialty titles in areas that will match your interests. You will be updated on what's new in books at no cost to you. Just fill in the coupon below and discover the convenience of having books delivered to your home.

PLEASE ADD $1.00 TO COVER THE COST OF POSTAGE & HANDLING.

BOOKS BY MAIL

320 Steelcase Road E.,
Markham, Ontario L3R 2M1

210 5th Ave., 7th Floor
New York, N.Y., 10010

Please send Books By Mail catalogue to:

Name _____
                    (please print)
Address _____

City _____

Prov./State _____ P.C./Zip _____

(BBM1)

WAYNE D. OVERHOLSER
WESTERNS

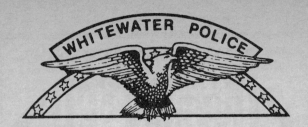

JOHN BALL
AUTHOR OF **IN THE HEAT OF THE NIGHT** INTRODUCING, **POLICE CHIEF JACK TALLON** IN THESE EXCITING, FAST-PACED MYSTERIES.

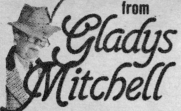